T0319633

Social Justice
and the
Urban Obesity Crisis

Social Justice and the Urban Obesity Crisis

Implications for Social Work

MELVIN DELGADO

Columbia University Press *New York*

Columbia University Press
Publishers Since 1893
New York   Chichester, West Sussex
cup.columbia.edu
Copyright © 2013 Columbia University Press
All rights reserved

Library of Congress Cataloging-in-Publication Data
Delgado, Melvin.
Social justice and the urban obesity crisis: implications for social works / Melvin Delgado.
pages cm
Includes bibliographical references and index.
ISBN 978-0-231-16008-7 (cloth: alk. paper)—ISBN 978-0-231-16009-4 (pbk.: alk. paper)—
ISBN 978-0-231-53425-3 (e-book)
1. Obesity—Social aspects.   I. Title.
RA645.O23D45 2013
362.1963'98—dc23
2012033984

Columbia University Press books are printed on permanent and durable acid-free paper.
This book is printed on paper with recycled content.
Printed in the United States of America

c 10 9 8 7 6 5 4 3 2 1
p 10 9 8 7 6 5 4 3 2 1

COVER PHOTO: © Paul Mounce / Corbis
COVER DESIGN: Milenda Nan Ok Lee

References to websites (URLs) were accurate at the time of writing. Neither the author nor
Columbia University Press is responsible for URLs that may have expired or changed since
the manuscript was prepared.

This book is dedicated to my spouse Denise,

a constant source of support,

and to my daughters Laura and Barbara,

constant sources of inspiration.

Contents

Acknowledgments

I want to acknowledge the contributions of Ms. Lyndsy Avalone and Ms. Cate Johnston, research assistants, Boston University School of Social Work. They worked tirelessly and provided important perspectives on the evolution of this book.

1

Setting the Context

1

Introduction

America is fat. For some, the evidence is readily apparent: a cavernous dent in the once-sturdy couch, the belt which grows like kudzu, the cruel reminders in the eyes of strangers. For others, though, the obesity epidemic is something troubling but external, alien even, like the neighbors two streets over who leave old car parts in their yard—best kept away from, or at the very least, complained about in the safety of similarly tasteful friends; a sign of personal collapse and failure best glowered over as a Washington Post editorial or chuckled at as a New Yorker cartoon.

(BENFORADO, HANSON, AND YOSIFON, 2006, P. 1645)

The opening quote captures a multitude of perspectives on the social phenomenon that we call *obesity*, a much-talked-about condition, judging by the amount of publicity and scholarly attention it has generated in recent decades. Is there a need for an entire book on overweight and obesity—specifically one premised on a social justice paradigm and aimed at the social work profession? I hope that this book will prove the answer to be a resounding *yes*.

At the outset it is important to define the terms *overweight* and *obesity* and to consider whether there truly is an obesity "epidemic." A look at media and scholarly treatments of the issue and a brief history of our changing attitudes toward weight will offer a context that will be useful. Other aspects of the inquiry will examine individual and environmental factors related to obesity, provide an overview of programs intended to combat this condition, discuss obesity's particular impact on urban communities of color, and explore the potential of social work for addressing this complicated health issue.

The subject of obesity will only increase in significance nationally and internationally in the immediate future (M. C. Smith, 2009). Social workers are in a unique position to make a significant contribution to the ongoing discourse (in research, scholarship, and practice) because of our embrace of social justice, our history of community practice, and our use of multi-intervention methods.

The World Health Organization's Commission on the Social Determinants of Health advocates for a policy agenda rooted in social epidemiology and human rights with direct relevance to overweight and obesity (Burris and Anderson, 2010). A social justice perspective represents a lens through which we can examine interventions that target obesity, while understanding the political reasons why certain population groups of this nation have a disproportionate chance of gaining excessive weight and are at higher risk for the many health conditions and complications that result.

Defining Overweight and Obesity

Defining what constitutes *overweight* and *obese* can be difficult, and some critics argue that any result of such an effort is socially constructed and highly politicized.

The standard measurement for excessive weight is determined by calculating the *body mass index* (BMI). This figure is determined by multiplying a person's weight in pounds by 703, and then dividing the resulting number by the square of the person's height in inches (Mantel, 2010). According to the National Institutes of Health, to be classified as overweight, women must have a BMI of 27.3 or higher, and men a BMI of 27.8 or higher. An individual is considered obese if he or she has a BMI of 30 or higher.

A 1999–2004 study of overweight and obesity in the United States found significant increases over the past several decades, and an alarming rate of increase (Ogden et al., 2006). Further, Strum (2007) found that between 2000 and 2008 the prevalence of *severe obesity* (individuals who weigh at least 100 pounds more than their recommended weight) increased two to three times faster than that of moderate obesity.

It should be noted when presenting these statistics that the field of obesity research faces broad challenges, as identified by Canay and Buchan (2007): (1) inaccurate and incomplete assessment of energy balance; (2) unclear implications of long-term excessive weight on health; (3) underestimation of obesity-related burden of disease; (4) poor understanding of childhood obesity; (5) inadequate study of population-level prevention measures and interventions; and (6) narrow scope of policy analysis. These six limitations will be addressed throughout this book.

How did we arrive at a point at which being overweight or obese can be considered normative? The journey took place over an extended period of time. The typical male adolescent in 2012 consumes 2,800 calories per day, an increase of 250 calories since the late 1970s; a typical female adolescent consumes 1,900, or an increase of 120 calories (Finkelstein and Zuckerman, 2008). Such seemingly small increases can add up to significant gains in weight: adding just 100 calories per day can translate into a gain of 10 pounds per year (Finkelstein and Zuckerman, 2008). Couple the increase in calories consumed with a reduction in exercise and take into account genetic factors (it is estimated that 70 percent of a person's body weight is the result of biological factors), and it becomes clear that it is a real challenge not to gain weight!

The prevalence of overweight and obesity is not confined to the United States; it is particularly evident among children living in urban centers of economically developed countries (Seidell, 2000; Wang and Lobstein, 2006; Waters et al., 2008). Bulgaria (Ivanova, Dimitrov, Dellava, and Hoffman, 2008), Canada (Elliott, 2010; Harrington and Elliott, 2009), Sweden (Neovius, Janson, and Rossner, 2006), China (Reynolds et al., 2007; Wu, 2006; Zhai et al., 2009), Latin America, and the Caribbean (Rueda-Clausen, Silva, and Lopez-Jaramillo, 2007), for example, report alarming trends of overweight and obesity. Developing countries, too, are coping with the paradox of obesity and malnutrition (Prentice, 2006).

By these definitions, the World Health Organization (2011) estimates that globally there are more than 1.5 billion overweight adults, at least 500 million of whom are obese (200 million men and 300 million women). This is more than every woman, man, and child in the United States being obese!

In discussing conditions of being obese, overweight, or, more commonly, fat, commentators in the media often use terms that Klein (2006) considers "biblical in their moral disapprobation." Kuczmarski (2007) notes that the term *obesity* is bound to elicit a wide range of reactions, depending upon a host of factors (including the knowledge base, experience, and background of the individual responding). Further compounding the confusion, the terms *overweight* and *obese* are often used interchangeably. The social consequences of these conditions can be quite distressing: being "fat" influences self-image, increases the likelihood of discrimination, and is also linked to lower economic status and poorer health outcomes.

Society often does not represent or seek the perspective of those who are overweight. Cooper (2009a) counteracts this omission by addressing the importance of upending society's tendency to stigmatize or demonize those who are overweight or obese. *Fat acceptance* or *"Fat-Lib"* efforts serve to empower those who are overweight or obese (Cooper, 2010).

Pomeranz (2008, p. S93) addresses the importance of legislation against weight bias but acknowledges the challenges in bringing such policies to fruition:

> History teaches that discrimination against socially undesirable groups leads to societal and governmental neglect of the stigmatized group's health problem. [Viewing] weight discrimination in a historical context . . . demonstrates that legislation specifically aimed at rectifying obesity is less likely while weight bias is socially acceptable. Beyond obesity legislation, public health professionals may consider advocating for legislation directly targeting discrimination based on weight.

Hopkins (2011) discusses how body size and shape (specifically overweight or obesity) negatively influence identity, the way individuals navigate through society, and the inequalities that they encounter. Sweeting (2011) comments on recent highly publicized actions that single out those who are obese, such as efforts to require that airline passengers who are obese pay for two seats rather than one seat.

Nevertheless, as Cooper (2009b, p. 1) notes, our bias toward "fat" people may even prevent us from recognizing the significance of an activist movement led by these individuals:

> In 21st century Western civilization, obesity is such a maligned state of being that the notion of fat activism is unthinkable within dominant obesity discourse. The lead of "activist" suggests a dynamic engagement with public life . . . that would not be further from couch potato stereotypes associated with fat people, or popular discourses which typify "the obese" through moral narratives as innately unwholesome, passive recipients of pity and intervention. Yet activism exists, has a complex history and offers new ways of conceptualizing "obesity."

Is There an Obesity "Epidemic"?

The term *epidemic* has been used countless times to describe the problem of overweight and obesity (Gilman, 2008). A 2007 Surgeon General's report, for example, officially labeled the problem an "epidemic." Some scholars question this usage, however. See, for example, Flegal (2006, p. 77): "The word 'epidemic' has some drawbacks as a descriptor. Because it has no quantitative definition, there is no precise way to determine whether something is an epidemic or not, and opinions may differ."

The term *epidemic* has a way of being used to draw attention to a particular situation or condition (Gilman, 2008). An article in the *Washington Times* (Duke, 2010) titled "'Epidemic' growth of the Net porn cited" is such an example. Another is Taylor (2009), "Fear of Failure: A Childhood Epidemic." A search of the literature will find the term associated with "crime," "sexual abuse," "autism," "depression," "sexually transmitted diseases," and "substance abuse." Klein (2006), as well as others, wonders why other widespread phenomena—automobile accidents or pollution, for example—are not considered epidemics? It seems as though there is no social condition or problem that cannot benefit from the label. However, there are economic and political forces at work that influence its use as a designation. Some question whether the term is overused by industries (such as the food, exercise, and diet industries) and interest groups (such as some in the scientific industry) that financially benefit directly from the "epidemic" label (Campos, 2004; Campos, Saguy, Ernsberger, Oliver, and Gaesser, 2006; Gibbs, 2005; Oliver, 2006). "Obesity Inc." has been the label assigned to these interests (Mundy, 2002).

Oliver (2006, p. 5) blames the usage on the scientific community:

> What I came to discover was that, contrary to the conventional wisdom, the primary source of America's obesity epidemic is not to be found at McDonald's, Burger King, or Krispy Kreme Donuts . . . or any of the other theories that are often used to explain our rising weights. Rather, America's obesity epidemic originates in far less conspicuous sources. The most important of these is America's public health establishments. Over the past two decades, a handful of scientists, doctors, and health officials have actively campaigned to define our growing weight as an "obesity epidemic."

Flegal (2006), however, argues that there is no escaping the high prevalence and rapid increase of overweight and obesity. McKinnon (2010, p. 309), sums up the gravity of this phenomenon: "Certain aspects of the obesity epidemic in the United States are not in question. We know, for instance, that rates of obesity (defined as BMI equal to or greater than 30) for all sociodemographic groups have risen to a startling degree in the past 50 years, and that 33.8 percent of U.S. adults are classified as obese, as are 16.9 percent of children."

Media and Scholarly Attention

The labeling of obesity as an epidemic has benefited from significant media and scholarly attention. Hardly a day goes by without a story in the national media about how Americans have progressively gotten heavier and as a result, unhealthier (Hill, Wyatt, Reed, and Peters, 2003; Kolata, 2011; Parikh et al., 2008). Kumanyika and Brownson (2007) discuss how media coverage of obesity conveys a perpetual national crisis, with dire predictions about the future of overweight individuals. Boero (2007) analyzed the *New York Times* between 1990 and 2001 and found 751 articles on obesity, many of which focused on individual instead of macro-level forces, making it more of a medicalized, or pathologized, phenomenon. Ten Eyck (2007) studied national newspaper sections devoted to food and fitness during a one-month period (August 2005) and found that the topic of obesity appeared in 592 articles.

Saguy (2005) found that from 1994 to 2004, the number of scholarly medical articles on obesity tripled, while those in the popular press quadrupled. In 2001, the number of media articles on obesity surpassed those on hunger, even though the World Health Organization labeled hunger as the primary cause of death in the world!

Saguy and Almeling (2008) concluded that the media exhibit a propensity to report more heavily on the most alarmist scientific studies, as well as on those that blame individual factors, to the exclusion of those that offer alternative explanations. (It should be noted that alternative theories are much more complex to report, and much more politically charged. An article that implicates food industry practices as an underlying cause of obesity, for example, may have ramifications for advertising revenues. After all, individuals rarely advertise in the media, but corporations do.)

The scientific community, not surprisingly, has also published extensively on the topic. For example, the journals *Future of Children* (Spring, 2006), *Science* (February, 2003), *Health Affairs* (March, 2010), and *International Journal of Epidemiology* (February, 2006) devoted special issues to obesity, and at least four scholarly journals are devoted solely to obesity (*International Journal of Pediatric Obesity; Obesity; Obesity Research*; and *Obesity Reviews*). This trend reveals the significant foothold that issues of overweight and obesity have gained among scholars.

Changing Attitudes Toward Weight: A Brief History

Gilman (2010), a social-cultural historian, shows how the meaning attached to the condition of obesity has evolved, from ancient Greece to the present day. His book *Fat: A Cultural History of Obesity* (2008) posits that our national obsession with "fat" is not new and can be traced back to the mid-nineteenth century.

Interestingly, the term *diet* has its roots in the Greek word *dioeta*. However, the original meaning, "a prescribed course of life," did not necessarily indicate an exclusive focus on food (Oliver, 2006). Gilman (2010) traces obesity as a pathological condition back to ancient Greece and Hippocrates (ca. 440–370 BCE).

Obesity in the eighteenth century was considered a condition of the wealthy (Gilman, 2010). It acquired a stigma only after it became associated with the lower classes. In the 1860s, William Banting, a formerly obese Englishman, published a pamphlet titled *Letter on Corpulence, Addressed to the Public*, which described the success of his diet and is considered the first publication on dieting (Greenblatt, 2003). Wolin and Petrelli (2009) note that by the turn of the nineteenth century, many Americans began to view excessive weight as socially undesirable. New inventions, such as portable scales (1891) and the first bathroom scale, the "Health-O-Meter" (1919), made it easier to keep track of weight gain. Levenstein (2003) discusses how from 1880 to 1930, new nutritional science theories and the rise of labor-saving food and devices radically altered the American diet.

Around this time, LuLu Hunt Peters published *Dieting and Health, with Key to the Calories* (1918), widely considered to be the first best-selling diet book in the United States (Gilman, 2010). Peters targeted women and framed obesity as a condition resulting from overindulgence, highlighting personal factors (such as a genetic resistance to gaining weight, or not having the skills to resist temptation) as the primary issues related to weight. The evolution of the diet industry from these humble beginnings to a $35 billion a year industry is history, so to speak. Stewart and

Korol (2009) note that the recognition of obesity as a serious health issue in the United States began around this time, when future president Herbert Hoover, then head of the U. S. Food Administration, introduced calorie counting. By the 1920s dieting was becoming an obsession among adolescent girls.

Sadly, the targeting of women by the diet industry has continued to evolve since then. In *The Female Eunuch* (1971), Germaine Greer highlighted how society has demanded that women be thin, often to the point that they become susceptible to eating disorders. Wiseman, Gray, Mosimann, and Aherns (1992) reported an overemphasis on diet and exercise articles in women's magazines during the period 1959–1988. More recently, a meta-analysis of 77 studies found that exposure to media images emphasizing thinness is positively associated with body image concerns among women (Grabe, Ward, and Hyde, 2008). The goal of achieving thinness is a critical element in bulimia nervosa among women (Chernyak and Lowe, 2010), resulting in a lucrative market of products and services addressing eating disorders (Hesse-Biber, Leavy, Quinn, and Zoino, 2006).

In the 1960s, weight and beauty ideals shifted once again: "Yet for reasons that are still unclear, in the early 1960s the beauty and fashion pendulum began to swing back toward the thin ideal. A statistical analysis of the measurements of Playboy centerfolds and Miss America pageant contestants in the 1960s and 1970s has charted this, showing how both groups of women became considerably thinner over that period" (Levenstein, 1993, p. 239). The early 1970s, however, also witnessed an increase in the number of books targeting the food industry's undermining of this nation's health (Levenstein, 1993).

Awareness about obesity prevention began to emerge in the mid-1990s with the publication of an article by Kuczmarski, Flegal, Campbell, and Johnson (1994) and a report by the National Task Force on Prevention and Treatment of Obesity (Kumanyika, 2007). An American Medical Association report (1999) that tied 300,000 annual deaths in the United States to obesity is also considered partially responsible for the upsurge in national media attention (Gibbs, 2005). In 2001 the surgeon general issued a report titled *A Surgeon General's Call to Action to Prevent and Reduce Overweight and Obesity*, which also increased governmental and media attention.

Any listing of current books on weight loss would be far too extensive to include here. To mention just a couple of examples, Dr. Phil, a well-known television personality with a reputation for addressing thorny personal problems, wrote *The Ultimate Weight Solution* (2003), which topped the *New York Times* best seller list, and Dr. Robert Atkins, a leading diet author, has sold more than 10 million copies of his books (Greenblatt, 2003).

One of the latest fad diets making the news as this book goes to press encourages the use of hCG (a pregnancy hormone), combined with a limited caloric intake (approximately 500 calories per day) to achieve weight loss without feeling tired and hungry (Hartocollis, 2011). However, like all "miracle" diets, this one brings with it Food and Drug Administration warnings regarding significant health risks.

Paradis (2010) commented on our current obsession with "fat" and the importance of understanding its social construction: "Over the past century, our culture's interest in fat has escalated dramatically. Be it nutritional fat, fat as a public health problem, fat as a financial burden, fat as a biological or hereditary trait, or fat as a social construction and cultural obsession, scholars from all disciplines have participated in defining what fat is, what it means, and why and how it matters."

Gilman (2008, p. 14) also commented on the evolution of our concern with overweight and obesity: "Obesity as a category has been the subject of . . . public reconceptualization over the past decades. It has become the target of public health campaigns and spurred a global rethinking of where the sources of danger for the public may lie. Such a rethinking mixes together and stirs many qualities in order to provide a compelling story that defines 'obesity' as the 'new public health epidemic.'"

Whose Problem Is It? Individual Versus Ecological Factors

Determining who is responsible for the problem of excessive weight goes a long way toward determining who should address it and how. Numerous strategies have been put forth for how best to address overweight and obesity. These strategies vary depending on whether one sees as the primary cause of excess weight (1) individual responsibility or (2) ecological factors (which include family, home, social and peer networks, the built environment, and community factors). Each of these approaches has its following, and each embraces a set of values and principles that guides assessment and corresponding interventions.

Individual Responsibility

What we eat, and how much we eat, is at the center of the discourse on individual responsibility. Mikkelsen, Erikson, Sims, and Nestle (2010, p. 292) address the role food plays within a sociocultural context: "Food is a unique component of life in that it provides the nutrition necessary for our health and survival while also playing a central role in the customs and traditions that add meaning to our lives. Although the need for food is fundamentally biological, we select our diets in the context of the social, economic, and cultural environments in which we live."

Food taps cultural customs and traditions as well as biological needs, all while influencing health—and therein lies the challenge and opportunity for social-work-focused community interventions. Eating is a basic human need, but what we eat is laden with deep symbolic meaning. Further, food is a commodity, and companies in the food industry are subject to pressure to maximize their market share and profit. Thus the constant bombardment of messages about the importance of being thin comes up against a similar, if not more powerful, bombardment of advertisements for foods that have limited health benefits and increase the likelihood of gaining weight. Given these competing messages, the average person faces a no-win situation. Steven N. Blair, quoted in Gibbs (2005, p. 77), notes: "We have got to stop shouting from the rooftops that obesity is bad for you and that fat people are evil and weak-willed and that the world would be lovely if we all lost weight. We need to take a much more comprehensive view. But I don't see much evidence that that is happening."

Dorfman and Wallack (2007, p. S45) summarize the debate over food choice from an individual versus an ecological perspective: "Currently, nutrition is described primarily as a matter of individual responsibility, which results in a focus on limited strategies that are unlikely to be successful. Public health advocates need to change the terms of debate or 'reframe' the issue so that the context around individuals—the social, economic, and political context—comes into view."

Ecological Factors

Dorfman and Wallack allude to significant ecological factors that can influence weight, such as severely limited food choices (resulting from lack of access and/or money) and an inability to engage in physical exercise in safe environments. Such environmental barriers can explain why some populations are at risk for excessive weight gain. These same populations also face incredible odds against their receiving quality health care to deal with the myriad health consequences and disparities associated with excessive weight.

Those who take an ecological perspective ask different questions, and subscribe to a different set of values, than do adherents of the individual responsibility school. Lawrence (2004) concludes that in recent years a systems perspective (one that sees obesity as a public health problem that is amenable to broad social policy initiatives) has emerged. Adherents of this perspective argue that the implications of excessive weight go far beyond health and can also be understood from economic, social, and, some would argue, political perspectives. In fact, a socioecological viewpoint is necessary to achieve a comprehensive understanding of the multifaceted forces at work to create the obesity epidemic.

A socioecological perspective helps us to understand the systematic, dynamic, and interactive aspects of overweight and obesity (DeMattia and Denney, 2008; Huberty, Balluff, O'Dell, and Peterson, 2010; Lee and Cubbin, 2009). It encourages development of strategies that focus on environments, such as policies promoting physical activity (Honisett, Woolcock, Porter, and Hughes, 2009), healthy diets for families (Warren, 2010), schools (Foster et al., 2008; Slusser, Cumberland, Browdy, Winham, and Neumann, 2005), child care centers (Fitzgibbon, Stolley, Schiffer, Horn, Christoffel, and Dyer, 2005; Ford, Veur, and Foster, 2007), and communities (McLaren, 2007), to list but a few.

As a more specific example, many who study the impact of environmental factors point to the practices of the food industry (sometimes referred to as "Big Food") as they influence overweight and obesity. Schlosser's (2005) hugely popular book *Fast Food Nation: The Dark Side of the All-American Meal* presented a disparaging picture of the fast-food industry and its impact on the nation, particularly on youth. Nestle's (2007) *Food Politics: How the Food Industry Influences Nutrition and Health* analyzed how the food industry, through lobbying, advertising, and undermining/co-opting experts, systematically protects its economic interests at the expense of the public's health. Simon (2006a) echoes a similar argument in *Appetite for Profit: How the Food Industry Undermines Our Health and How to Fight Back*. These and other books have challenged the food industry and its role in causing and sustaining the obesity crisis in this country and globally.

The food industry's response to these accusations has been multifaceted (Nestle, 2007; Simon, 2006b; Wansink and Peters, 2007): (1) deny any malicious role in creating the crisis; (2) argue about individual consumer responsibility; (3) lobby for "Commonsense Consumption" laws that exempt the industry from any civil liability concerning overweight and obese customers; (4) redouble efforts at lobbying of third parties; (5) sponsor industry-backed scientific research; and (6) develop a "win-win" strategy. The fifth point can be illustrated by clever marketing of new packaging, for example: "Take the notion of single-serving packaging. Although such packaging would increase production costs, the $40 billion spent each year on diet-related products is evidence that there is a portion-predisposed segment that would be willing to pay a premium for packaging that enabled them to eat less of a food in a single serving and to enjoy it more" (Wansink and Peters, 2007, p. 195).

Advocates of the food industry are quick to argue that it can, and does, exercise self-regulation. However, critics point to its lobbying and deceptive practices as evidence that it cannot self-regulate, with the federal government exercising minimal oversight, and complicit university scientists providing industry-sponsored research attesting to numerous "facts" about the nutritional value and effectiveness of food products resulting in weight loss (Nestle, 2007; Simon, 2006b).

Obviously, the answer to how best to address excessive weight depends upon who is asking the question and formulating the analysis (Benforado et al., 2006, p. 1652):

> Facing up to the fact that obesity in America is *our* problem, whether we are six-pack crunchers or six-pack guzzlers, gets us only so far. The issues of causation remain. Only recently have scientists begun to sort through the genetic, behavioral, and environmental factors that have a direct impact on body weight. Although the evidence remains hotly contested, especially by fast-food companies facing potential liability, the emerging consensus among public health experts is that obesity is largely a product of a "toxic environment."

The term *toxic environment*, similar to *obesogenic environment*, stresses how the powerful socioecological influence of where we live can undermine our efforts at achieving good health, such as by avoiding excessive weight.

Individual and Ecological Factors

Ultimately, the latest research suggests that obesity results from a complex interplay between individual and environmental components. There may be a genetic cause that is "triggered" by lifestyle or environmental factors.

The topic of genetics is far beyond the scope of this book. Much progress has been made in the past several years to identify genes associated with excessive weight. In fact, scientists have discovered 17 single-nucleotide polymorphisms (the most common form of genetic variation among humans) that wield an influence on obesity. One gene in particular, the fat mass and obesity-associated protein FTO, is responsible for 22 percent of obesity cases (Mantel, 2010). FTO is believed to operate in the regions of the brain that regulate appetite and satiety.

Nevertheless, a biological predisposition toward excessive weight gain is best conceptualized along a continuum (Mantel, 2010). In essence, there is a predisposition, or individual susceptibility, toward excessive weight (James, Jackson-Leach, and Rigby, 2010). Environmental factors, in turn, heighten or diminish the probability of gaining or losing weight.

In this sense, there are similarities with certain forms of cancer that are more likely to occur because of lifestyle choices. The correlation between cigarette smoking and lung cancer is one obvious example, but not everyone who smokes cigarettes is guaranteed to develop lung cancer. The causes of cancer are quite complex. So, too, are the causes of overweight and obesity.

Ulijaszek (2008) identified six models of population obesity, each having profound implications for assessment and intervention: (1) thrifty genotypes (a biological ability to fatten during periods of abundance, which aids survival during periods of famine); (2) obesogenic behavior (behaviors, such as lack of physical activity and excessive media viewing, that may lead to weight gain); (3) obesogenic environments (environmental influences that encourage excessive caloric intake); (4) nutrition transition (increased consumption of unhealthy foods); (5) obesogenic culture (a cultural valuing of obesity as a sign of wealth and success); and (6) biocultural interactions of genetics, environment, behavior, and culture.

Because of the numerous factors that influence weight, the study of overweight and obesity can draw upon the sociology of the body (the study of images and social uses of the human body), moral panic theory (intensity of feelings about a particular issue resulting in a threat to societal values), and critical weight studies (a focus on how obesity is acted upon by the media and key institutions drawing attention to the consequences of excessive weight), for example, to more fully increase our understanding of this phenomenon (Cohen, 2003; Laqueur, 1999; Rich, Monaghan, and Aphramor, 2011). Examining these factors in isolation from contextual forces and demography, however, serves only to further negate the role of other environmental forces that are oppressive in character.

Obesity and Urban Communities of Color

I realize that obesity is a nationwide phenomenon that can be found in all communities, urban and rural, privileged and non-privileged. The problem of overweight and obesity reaches into all major demographic sectors of society. However, it has a particular impact on those sectors that are the most marginalized or undervalued because of lack of income and wealth, and race/ethnicity. Those sectors are also the most likely to experience significant health disparities because of limited access to quality health care. Consequently, although overweight and obesity are serious national problems, it is my contention, and that of many other practitioners and academics, that these problems are particularly acute in undervalued urban communities (Committee on Health Care for Underserved Women, 2010; Trent, Jennings, Waterfield, Lyman, and Thomas, 2009).

According to the Office of Minority Health (2011 a, b, c, d, e), people of color face disproportionately greater consequences related to obesity because its prevalence is so high in their communities. Among Native Hawaiians/Pacific Islanders, 63.5 percent of all adults 18 years and older are obese; among American Indian/Alaska Natives, 34 percent; African Americans/Blacks, 33 percent; Latinos, 31.7 percent; and Asian Americans, 12.5 percent. These statistics do not include obesity rates among children and youth, which further compound the problem of overweight and obesity in communities of color.

That is why this book focuses on those communities (Corburn, 2009, p. 2): "American cities—or more precisely certain neighborhoods in these cities—are facing a health crisis. While not a new phenomenon, the urban poor, immigrants and people of color die earlier and suffer more, by almost every measure of disease, than any population group in the United States."

The United States Department of Agriculture (2009) estimated that in 2008 17.1 million families in the United States experienced food insecurity (lack of financial resources to purchase enough food). Further, these families also had the highest rates of poverty, obesity, and diabetes (Drewnowski and Specter, 2004). These families, however, were not evenly distributed across all regions of the country. Major urban areas accounted for a disproportionate number of families facing food shortages and also combating excessive rates of obesity and other weight-related illnesses.

The consequences of overweight and obesity are also particularly severe in urban marginalized communities because of a host of social-environmental forces (Corburn, 2009; Drewnowski, Rehm, and Solet, 2007; Marmot and Wilkinson, 2006). (The term *marginalized* is used in this book to characterize specific groups, such as those who have low income, are of color, and/or are living in urban communities where they represent a high percentage of the population. Other terms used in this book include *communities of color* or *people of color*, my preferred terminology for racial and ethnic groups—typically African Americans, Asians, and Latinos—that are often referred to as "minorities." These groups, however, consist of multiple subgroups from different countries of origin and are not monolithic in structure and composition.) The consequences of overweight and obesity when combined with a host of factors that limit access to healthy foods and physical exercise can be deadly.

In addition, sub-population groups such as women, children, and older adults will be highlighted because of their particular vulnerability regarding overweight and obesity (Adler and Stewart, 2009; Black and Macinko, 2007). Howe, Patel, and Galobardes (2010, p. 404) state this point succinctly:

Obesity is concentrated in the most deprived sections of the community in most high-income countries in both adults and children. This is also increasingly true of low- and middle-income countries (where historically the inequality has operated in the opposite direction), particularly amongst women. Diet and physical activity and their socio-economic patterning are likely to be affected by individual factors, local social context (including family, peers, workplace, and community), and by wider societal influences (such as food pricing and availability, provision of facilities for physical activity, welfare state policies and so on).

Anti-Obesity Policies and Programs

Government Programs

The role of government (federal, state, and local) should be to promote the health and well-being of all its citizens. In pursuing that goal, government can be influential in reducing, and even preventing, overweight and obesity, as witnessed in Australia, Sweden, and other parts of the world (Haire-Joshu, Fleming, and Schermbeck, 2007). The government's role, however, must go beyond the issuing of reports and the raising of public consciousness.

Haire-Joshu, Fleming, and Schermbeck (2007) identified six key tasks that the federal government can undertake in this effort: (1) funding research; (2) fostering services that target the highest-risk population groups; (3) supporting nutritional and physical activity programming at the community-level; (4) assessing and developing relevant surveillance and monitoring efforts; (5) promoting healthy diets and physical activity; and (6) sponsoring and evaluating projects that promote healthy diets and physical activity. Funding for these types of initiatives, however, has suffered in the current economic downturn, with profound implications for the population groups hardest hit by the crisis.

Despite this, numerous programs at the federal level have sought to address overweight and obesity. In 2010 President Obama established the White House Task Force on Childhood Obesity. Obama also proclaimed September 2010 as the first Childhood Obesity Awareness Month, as another way of increasing public awareness of the problem for children. Michelle Obama's child-focused "Let's Move" campaign received significant economic stimulus funding (Martin, 2009). In early 2011 she launched a program to encourage restaurants to offer smaller portions and to include healthier options in children's meals (Stolberg and Neuman, 2011).

Unfortunately, many federal anti-obesity activities have focused on individual responsibility and have left industries free to continue their practices without fear of retribution. For example, there have been a number of efforts to pass federal legislation to shield the industry from lawsuits. These efforts have been labeled as "personal responsibility," "frivolous lawsuits," and "cheeseburger bills," as a way of shaming anyone who sees merit in using the legal system to curb industry practices (Simon, 2006b). Pomeranz (2008, p. 96) examines congressional testimony and state hearings and highlights quotes that attempt to blame individuals and absolve the industry:

- "This bill is about self-responsibility. If you eat too much, you get fat. It is your fault. Don't try to blame somebody else."
- "It is clear that obesity is a problem in America. Equally clear, however, is that ample availability of high-fat food is not a singular or even a primary cause."
- "The victim always finds someone else to blame for his or her own behavior. And what this bill does is that it says, do not run off and file a lawsuit if you are too fat and you end up getting the diseases associated with obesity. It says, look in the mirror, because you are the one who is to blame."

Between 2003 and 2006, 24 states enacted legislation protecting fast-food establishments from liability, reflecting the sentiment that when it comes to the unhealthy consequences of fast food, "let the buyer beware" (Pomeranz, 2008).

Consider recent campaigns against sugary drinks as another example. It is estimated that the average American has doubled his or her intake of sugar-sweetened beverages over the past thirty years (Mantel, 2010). This increase translates into 175 calories per day per person—or potentially 18 additional pounds per year (Mantel, 2010). In response, a number of high-profile organizations—including the American Academy of Pediatrics, the American Public Health Association, and the Institute of Medicine—have suggested that sweetened drinks be taxed, thereby making them more expensive to purchase and thus reducing consumption (Allday, 2010; Bittman, 2010; Douglas and Jacobson, 2010). However, the beverage industry has lobbied against such measures, somewhat successfully, as evidenced by New York State's failure to pass a proposed law (Hartocollis, 2010). Simon (2006a, pp. 287–288) draws an interesting conclusion about these industry efforts:

Industry's high powered lobbying effort is actually about much more than just passing bills. A convenient side effect of this lobbying crusade is to apply corporate spin to maximize effect. The rhetoric surrounding the lobbying shapes the broader debate related to who is to blame for obesity and diet-related health problems. Because lawsuits are such a hot-button issue, industry can take full advantage of the popular scapegoating of trial lawyers, while at the same time invoke all-American values and shove the personal responsibility theory down the nation's collective throat.

Burnett (2006–2007) critiques the efforts of Congress to ban fast-food lawsuits as misdirected and calls on Congress to focus on obesity as a major public health problem. Obesity and its consequences should be placed alongside the economy and national defense in any discussion of the national political agenda. Relegating this problem to secondary status undermines national attention and efforts at addressing the complexity of excessive weight in general, and in marginalized communities in particular.

Community Efforts

Many experts have begun to propose campaigns and programs that can have an impact on obesity on the community level. One promising strategy, for example, recommends that local governments offer economic incentives for attracting supermarkets to underserved communities (Mantel, 2010). Supermarkets, it should be noted, have a greater selection of healthy food at lower prices than do grocery and convenience stores (Khan et al., 2009).

Vallianatos (2009) offers a comprehensive vision for Los Angeles that has applicability for other urban centers and highlights a range of possible interventions that, when combined, offer hope for these communities. This vision is comprehensive, community-based, and predicated upon an in-depth understanding of current efforts across the country: (1) introduction of food vendors; (2) farmers' markets; (3) expansion of food retail outlets (smaller supermarkets); (4) nutrition labeling in restaurants; (5) fast-food restaurant moratorium; (6) more and better grocery stores; and (7) conversion of corner stores (incentives to sell more fruits and vegetables since they are lower-profit items).

Freudenberg, Bradley, and Serrano (2009) analyzed 12 campaigns intended to change industry practices that damage health (including the alcohol, automobile, food and beverage, firearms, pharmaceutical, and tobacco industries). They found that local campaigns were more effective in achieving change goals than national campaigns. In essence, all politics are local.

More specifically, the Centers for Disease Control and Prevention (Khan et al., 2009) identified 24 strategies that were supported by research and held significant promise for addressing obesity within a community context.

The Role of Social Work in Addressing Obesity

The multifaceted nature of this problem makes it imperative that all helping professions define and address it (Evangelista, Ortiz, Rios-Soto, and Urdapilleta, 2004). As already noted, hundreds, if not thousands, of articles have been written on overweight and obesity from a variety of disciplines. However, the field of social work has generally been silent on this issue, allowing other professions to conceptualize and address it. Social work has not contributed in any significant manner, even though the issues of healthy eating, overweight, and obesity are of tremendous importance, particularly in the lives of marginalized groups in this society.

The lack of coverage in the social work literature underscores the general oversight of overweight and obesity from a social work perspective. This does not mean that social workers are not involved in this field; major social work organizations have issued a charge for the profession to tackle obesity as part of health disparities, for example (Bywater, 2007). However, broad health-related charges to the profession do not emphasize the specific threat of excessive weight, and this problem often gets lost in the constellation of other health-related problems that social workers address.

The challenge of overweight and obesity necessitates a multidisciplinary approach at the macro, mezzo, and micro levels (Townshend, Ells, Alvanides, and Lake, 2010). The ability of social work to view this problem from individual, family, group, community, and policy perspectives is unprecedented in any other helping profession, and this breadth provides us with the ability to develop interventions founded on social justice principles (Donaldson and Daughtery, 2011; Kaiser, 2011).

Social work's embrace of a social justice paradigm encourages social workers to engage in social change campaigns that are centered in participatory democratic principles. The National Association of Social Workers (NASW) *Code of Ethics* (2008) specifically addresses the promotion of social justice and social change in all aspects of social work practice, stressing the needs and empowerment of people who are most vulnerable, oppressed, and living in poverty. Dorfman and Wallack (2007) call for the reframing of obesity and nutrition from an individual focus to one that is contextually (social, economic, and political) informed. Mitchell (2003) argues that one of the fundamental aspects of social justice is the advancement of a framework that stresses full and effective participation in the decision-making process by marginalized groups to address pressing concerns in their lives.

Studies and interventions on obesity often focus on individuals (Teufel-Shone, 2006) and on the importance of proper diet and exercise (Connelly, Duaso, and Butler, 2009; Spear et al., 2007). This perspective clearly lacks a social justice lens that an ecological perspective would bring. For example, park-based exercise programs targeting inner-city children and youth of color have found success when they take into account safety fears and crime (Bush et al., 2007). Similarly, Cutts, Darby, Boone, and Brewis (2009) found that Latinos and African Americans in Phoenix lived in walkable neighborhoods with access to parks, yet safety concerns prevented many residents from walking. Byrne, Wolch, and Zhang (2009) analyzed the Santa Monica Mountains National Recreation Area in Los Angeles and found that the nation's largest urban park, intended to attract urban residents of color, failed to do so by being perceived as unsafe from a psychological, rather than a physical, perspective. Perceptions, as a result, represent a dimension that must be addressed to encourage participation. Similarly, Gordon-Larsen, Nelson, Page, and Popkins (2006) found that low-income adolescents of color had limited access to physical activity facilities when compared with adolescents who were white, non-Latino, and had a higher SES. Thus, potential benefits of a *built environment* (which refers to urban design, land use, and transportation systems) intended to encourage physical activity can be negated by social circumstances such as crime and street violence.

Social Work and Health Promotion

Health promotion refers to interventions that seek to improve health and prevent or minimize the health consequences resulting from diseases and illnesses. It embraces a set of values, principles, theories, and methods that are influenced by social ecology and that view the individual in the context of his or her environment; thus they are resonant with social work. The field of health promotion experienced a tremendous surge in interest during the first decade of the twenty-first century as a result of increased governmental and scholarly attention (McQueen and Jones, 2007). In part, this occurred because issues of health are being analyzed in social, economic, and political terms (Cockerham, 2007).

This worldview takes on added significance when addressing the needs of population groups that are at increased risk for illness because of their marginalized social and economic status. The attention to health disparities, inequities, and inequalities is a testament to the importance of viewing health from a broad community or population perspective, rather than focusing on individuals. For instance, Kumanyika (2005) addresses health disparities and obesity in African American women and girls:

> The obesity prevalence data for black women are, by now, all too familiar. Seventy-seven percent of black women are in the overweight or obese (defined as having a body mass index [BMI] ≥25 kg/m^2) range, and 50% are in the obese range (BMI ≥30). . . . . The variation in obesity with socioeconomic status (SES) must be considered when comparing blacks and whites, but the higher obesity prevalence in black than white women is seen at all levels of typical SES indicators such as education and income. . . . The problem is not confined to adults. Among black girls, the high prevalence of obesity is of relatively recent onset but seems to have caught up with and passed the prevalence of obesity among white girls.

Reliance on a medical model, which historically has focused on individual lifestyle factors to the exclusion of environmental factors, prevents a multifaceted understanding of the factors leading to overweight and obesity. In addition, treatment is also individually focused (Adler and Stewart, 2009). A health promotion perspective broadens our understanding and approaches to combating this problem. When health promotion, in turn, adopts a social justice set of values and principles (predicated upon participatory democratic principles), these interventions can change the environmental circumstances that help cause overweight and obesity.

Social work, unfortunately, has not played a leadership role in developing health promotion strategies; yet we bring a profound understanding of communities, social ecology, social justice, and social interventions (Delgado and Zhou, 2008). Social work's absence, I believe, has done a disservice to the field of overweight and obesity. This book highlights the contributions that social work can make in the development of health promotion strategies targeting the problem of overweight and obesity in the United States.

Goals of This Book

This book seeks to discuss and promote promising community-based and -initiated strategies that address obesity and overweight in urban communities of color, using a social justice perspective, and with social work playing an active role in these interventions. As a result, this book seeks to accomplish six goals:

1. Provide readers with a state-of-the-art understanding of the magnitude and consequences of overweight and obesity in the United States.
2. Utilize a social justice perspective as a guide for assessing and addressing overweight and obesity in marginalized urban communities of color.
3. Focus specifically on the social causes and consequences among low-income urban groups of color, which are often the nation's fastest-growing demographic groups.
4. Examine the challenges in measuring the extent of the problem and achieving and evaluating intervention success.
5. Identify promising community-based participatory health promotion principles and interventions.
6. Identify how the profession of social work can play a prominent role in shaping overweight and obesity health promotion interventions.

To accomplish these goals I draw upon the latest literature, research, and thinking on the subject of overweight and obesity, nationally and internationally. Further, to make the book more reader-friendly, I present in-depth case examples, as well as shorter vignettes throughout the text.

2

A Social Justice Paradigm

Discrimination against stigmatized groups perpetuates the disparities prevalent in their lives. These disparities are not addressed appro-
priately by the government unless political support can be galvanized,
which has been historically difficult for socially disadvantaged groups.
Historically, those in power have advocated education and separation
as a solution to the health problems of stigmatized groups—neither of
which actually addresses the cause of increased incidence of disease
and both of which [result] in increased discrimination.

(POMERANZ, 2008, P. S94)

The reader may be puzzled by the introduction of a social justice paradigm so prominently in the title of a book about what is considered to
be a physical condition related to excessive food intake and a sedentary
lifestyle. What does weight have to do with social justice? The above quote
by Pomeranz (2008) explains why social justice plays such an important
role in this book and why social work must play an active role in dealing
with obesity.

Freeman's (2007, pp. 2221–2222) description of West Oakland, California, a community consisting primarily of low-income people of color,
illustrates the significance of social justice in addressing overweight and
obesity: "[West Oakland] has one supermarket and thirty-six liquor and
convenience stores. The supermarket is not accessible on foot to most
of the area's residents. The convenience stores charge twice as much as
grocery stores for identical items. Fast food restaurants selling cheap and
hot food appear on almost every corner. West Oakland is not unique." Indeed, this same description could apply to countless urban communities
across the country. A social justice perspective can analyze and explain
why West Oakland and other communities like it are so lacking in healthy
food options.

A social justice construct emphasizes the importance of justice for population groups and communities, and not just for individuals; as a result, it lends itself to broad-based analysis and interventions (Braithwaite, 2008; Schlosberg, 2007). A social justice perspective focused on equal distribution of rewards and burdens is very much a part of the social work *Code of Ethics* (Hoefer, 2006), further reinforcing the importance of viewing obesity and overweight in marginalized communities within this context.

This chapter lays out an in-depth argument for using social justice as a guiding paradigm in assessing and addressing overweight and obesity in undervalued communities in the United States, communities that tend to be predominantly low-income/low-wealth, urban, and of color. The argument proceeds through an analysis of social justice movements and obesity, a comparison of individual perspectives and social justice perspectives, and a discussion of food justice, environmental justice, and spatial justice as three interrelated issues that affect overweight and obesity. Finally it looks at health promotion programs that utilize a social justice framework and identifies the issues in evaluating the effectiveness of such programs.

Social Justice Movements and Obesity

Social movements invariably appear in response to an injustice of some kind that systematically singles out a specific group for oppression (Schlosberg, 2007, p. 39): "Social movements arise as responses to disrespect and misrecognition move from the individual and personal to the collective community." Social movements can also be conceptualized as a form of "collective struggles to achieve recognition" (Honneth, 1995, p. 164). Communities, which can be defined on the basis of shared geography, shared characteristics, or shared challenges, may develop a shared conception of what constitutes social injustice and how to redress the situation. In the case of this book, that conception revolves around the forces that lead to overweight and obesity through a focus on food, environment, or spatial justice (Schlosberg, 2007).

Tracing the origins of social justice movements is not easy: "Social movements are complex social constructions whose very existence as discriminable phenomena is frequently contested and sometimes unrecognized by the actors who participate in them, Indeed, the social scientist may, with the advantage of distance, theoretical perspective and conceptual apparatus, detect the existence of a social movement when all the actors can see is a confusion of organizations, campaigns and conflicts" (Rootes and Saunders, 2008, p. 1).

Kwan (2008) suggests three cultural frames for evaluating overweight and obesity: (1) medical (i.e., governmental agencies as represented by the Centers for Disease Control and Prevention); (2) market choice (industry); and (3) social justice (activists). Each of these cultural frames results in a different assessment of this social phenomenon, and consequently takes a different approach to addressing it. Each of the frames also subscribes to a set of values that shapes not only its perspective but also the terms used to describe the problem. A medical approach emphasizes the individual; a market choice, too, emphasizes personal choice and individuals. A social justice perspective is a natural extension of social work efforts at changing social structures and the forces that operate to perpetuate oppression in this society. This perspective emphasizes the importance of groups.

Individual Versus Social Justice Perspectives

Two perspectives are frequently used to blame the individual for his or her weight predicament: (1) that obesity is the result of lifestyle choices or (2) that obesity is a highly stigmatized state of being at the extreme end of the weight continuum (Puhl and Heuer, 2010; Ten Eyck, 2007). The latter is conceptualized by scholars who emphasize that "fat" people are discriminated against in all facets of life. The former is captured by Simon (2006b) in summarizing the food industry's strategies: "It is your fault you are in poor health because you have made poor decisions on food consumption, have failed to keep informed, and have failed to remain physically fit!"

Allen and Sachs (2007, p. 11) note how this message implicates mothers, in particular, when their children are overweight or obese: "Mothers often take the blame for their failure to provide their children with nutritious foods. Women with children are caught in a double bind as they are enjoined to make their children happy by feeding them junk food while they are simultaneously exhorted to be 'good mothers' by ensuring the nutritional health of their children."

Similarly, Brownell (2007, p. 116) highlights a paradox in personal responsibility:

At the heart of the consumer experience is a dominating paradox, one that strikes to the heart of what causes obesity and who is responsible for the solution. . . . At the same time individuals face a "toxic" or "obesogenic" environment that undermines personal responsibility and guarantees rising prevalence, people are blamed for their weight, face discrimination by virtue of being stigmatized, and are expected to prevail over the environment no matter how unhealthy it becomes.

Shifting thinking away from personal responsibility is a challenging task. When asked about the primary causes of obesity in a national survey, 71 percent of respondents attributed it to laziness, 20 percent mentioned unhealthy foods, and 9 percent mentioned genetics (Oliver, 2006). However, past efforts at interventions focused on individuals have met with very limited success, necessitating a shift toward communities and the forces that affect them (Barusch, 2009; Cummins and Macintyre, 2008).

Dorfman and Wallack (2007, p. S46) comment on how the food industry benefits from an individualized focus:

The food industry benefits when the focus is on obesity, because the way obesity is typically framed puts the blame on the person with the problem. The food and beverage industry can blame people's inability to control themselves and argue that problem "users," not problem products or problem promotions, cause obesity. The argument is akin to the way the alcohol industry benefits if the public focuses on alcoholics rather than the broad spectrum of alcohol problems.

Brownell and colleagues (2010, p. 379) sum up the weaknesses of the personal responsibility argument thus:

The concept of personal responsibility has been central to social, legal, and political approaches to obesity. It evokes language of blame, weakness, and vice and is a leading basis for inadequate government efforts, given the importance of environmental conditions in explaining high rates of obesity. These environmental conditions can override individual physical and psychological regulatory systems that might otherwise stand in the way of weight gain and obesity, hence undermining personal responsibility, narrowing choices, and eroding personal freedoms.

Brownell (2007, 117) also indicts the food industry for its reliance on the individual responsibility argument: "The U.S. food industry, its trade association and 'scientific' advisory groups, conservative political groups, shadow organizations masquerading as consumer groups, and political allies of these organizations are aggressive in pushing this responsibility position." Personal choices or responsible behavior can best be achieved in a supportive environment rather than in one that is toxic (Story, Kaphingst, Robinson-O'Brien, and Glanz, 2008).

In contrast to the personal responsibility position, Adler and Stewart (2009, p. 50) advance the concept of "behavioral justice" as means of connecting individual responsibility with forces that are outside individual control: "A social justice perspective facilitates a synthesis of both models. This article proposes the concept of 'behavioral justice' to convey the principle that individuals are responsible for engaging in health-promoting behaviors but should be held accountable only when they have adequate resources to do so. This perspective maintains both individuals' control and accountability for behaviors and society's responsibility to provide health-promoting environments."

A social justice paradigm provides social workers with a way of looking at obesity that emphasizes how social forces systematically target certain groups and communities because of their socio-demographic characteristics. A deficit, or personal responsibility, paradigm is thus countered, and instead the discourse can be shaped sociopolitically.

Some critics would go so far as to argue that a social justice paradigm, and the values it embraces, effectively politicizes what is essentially a "medical" condition. I would argue that it does just that, and rightly so! The subject of health does not exist in a social vacuum and cannot be divorced from social justice when focused on marginalized communities in this country (Buhin and Vera, 2009).

Powers and Faden, in *Social Justice: The Moral Foundation of Public Health and Health Policy* (2006), stress the importance of utilizing a social justice paradigm for understanding and addressing health disparities in this country. A social justice contextualization of health unites a seemingly disparate group of individuals under one sociopolitical umbrella. "Findings challenge health researchers and practitioners to understand health problems and health promotion not only at the individual level, but at multiple levels of influence including interpersonal, family, neighborhood, and structural levels" (de Jesus, 2009, p. 90).

Food Justice, Environmental Justice, and Spatial Justice

A social justice perspective regarding overweight and obesity in marginalized communities will be conceptualized in terms of three separate but complementary approaches here: (1) food justice (Wekerle, 2004); (2) environmental justice (Schlosberg, 2007; Wallace, 2008); and (3) spatial justice (Brown, Griffis, Hamilton, Irish, and Kanouse, 2007; Harris and Hooper, 2004). These three perspectives bring together into one analysis the key driving forces behind the increase in overweight and obesity in low-income urban communities of color.

Food Justice

The *food justice movement* evolved out of a growing concern that the global food system is unsustainable and unjust (Levkoe, 2006) and out of concerns about our overreliance upon standardized food created by industrialization (Hinrichs and Allen, 2008). This trend, some argue, has stripped food of its most basic value, which is to nurture both body and soul, and has profound implications for health. The consequences have been most severely felt in marginalized communities, which can ill afford poor nutrition.

The food justice movement encompasses a wide variety of efforts to secure food, and involves social action focused on creating a just food system (Levkoe, 2006). Terms such as *food democracy, food citizenship, food sovereignty, food security,* and *food sustainability*, for example, typify some of the more popular descriptions of this movement (Hansen, 2008; Hess, 2009; Kaiser, 2011; Renzaho and Mellow, 2009; Travaline, 2008). The movement is predicated on the belief that every person deserves healthy food, while assuming an equal distribution of risks and benefits associated with providing that food for all populations (Vallianatos, 2009). In essence, no one sector of the population should be saddled with poor nutrition while other sectors enjoy the benefits of healthy food.

Adherents of the food justice movement argue that there needs to be a reconceptualization of how individuals view their role and rights with relation to food. Wilkins (2007, p. 269) advances the concept of "food citizen" as a way of shifting our mind-set from thinking about individuals as consumers to thinking about them as people with rights and privileges: "The term food citizenship is defined as the practice of engaging in food-related behaviors that support, rather than threaten, the development of a democratic, socially and economically just, and environmentally sustainable food system."

Wilkins warns, however, that this shift will not be easy and must surmount four key barriers: (1) the current food system; (2) federal government food and agricultural policy; (3) local and institutional policies; and (4) the pervasive culture of professional nutrition organizations. Because its implications could significantly affect the way corporations produce, market, and sell food, the food justice movement has the potential to alter power relations between corporations and communities (Holt-Giménez and Shattuck 2011).

Maloni and Brown (2006) view social justice and the food industry from multiple perspectives: animal welfare, biotechnology, environment, fair trade, labor and human rights, health, and safety. They take a comprehensive view and argue that virtually all aspects of our daily lives are influenced by the food industry. Similarly, in 1996 the World Health Organization held the World Food Summit, which emphasized the interconnections between food and health, community economic development, environment, and trade.

The profit motive is the primary goal that drives this industry, and profit is maximized through promotion of foods with a high sugar and fat content, which are readily available, tasty, and inexpensive (Wansink and Peters, 2007). Caraher and Covency (2004) suggest that the global food market is controlled by a relatively small group of companies that essentially operate to provide "cheap" (energy-dense, micronutrient-poor) foods with little concern about nutritional value. These foods, in turn, find their way into undervalued communities (Swinburn, Caterson, Seidell, and James, 2004). Further, these foods bring store owners a high profit margin, making it attractive for local stores to advertise and stock them. A New Orleans study, for example, found that a typical neighborhood store derives a greater percentage of gross profits from snack foods and beverages than from fruits and vegetables (Bodor, Ulmar, Dunaway, Farley, and Rose, 2010).

Another explanation for the overabundance of unhealthy foods is government agricultural subsidies, particularly those offered for corn and soybean crops, which help to keep the costs of certain foods artificially low (Greenblatt, 2003). Subsidies make these crops more profitable to grow than other fruits and vegetables, and the resulting foods are less expensive to produce and sell (Finkelstein and Zuckerman, 2008).

These practices help to explain a seeming contradiction: the "paradox of plenty" (Nestle, 2007). There are more than one billion people in the world who suffer from starvation, and more than one billion who are overweight (New Economics, 2010). How can food abundance and starvation coexist? Consider Finkelstein and Zuckerman (2008, p. 31): "Truly, we live in a country that is rife with abundance. But here's the dilemma. Given the 'value' of cheap, tasty, super-size-portioned, calorie-dense foods, it's becoming increasingly difficult to maintain a healthy weight."

Nestle agrees (2007, p. 1): "The food industry has given us a food supply so plentiful, so varied, so inexpensive, and so devoid of dependence on geography or season that all but the poorest of Americans can obtain enough energy and nutrients to meet biological needs. Indeed, the U.S. food supply is so abundant that it contains enough to feed everyone in the country nearly twice over—even after exports are considered."

Altering a food system's production and distribution, while increasing food knowledge (McCullum, Desjardins, Kraak, Ladipo, and Costello, 2005), then becomes a central goal in a food justice approach toward reducing obesity. Current conventional food systems encourage unhealthy eating practices and limit, or restrict, access to healthy fruits and vegetables in marginalized neighborhoods (Powell, Slater, Mirtcheva, Bao, and Chaloupka, 2007; Taylor, Carlos Poston, Jones, and Kraft, 2006). The importance of healthy food production, accessibility, and fair pricing represents a critical social justice agenda when developing comprehensive strategies in urban communities if overweight and obesity are to be prevented or controlled.

Many states have started to recognize the limited access that certain communities have to supermarkets and affordable fresh fruits and vegetables (Treuhaft and Karpyn, 2011). A 2009 U.S. Department of Agriculture study found that 23.5 million people lacked physical access to a supermarket within one mile of their home (Treuhaft and Karpyn, 2011). It is estimated that in the United States there is one supermarket for every 8,000 residents, but some cities, such as Houston, have only one store per

12,000 residents (*Houston Chronicle*, 2011). Lack of ready access to supermarkets increases the likelihood of residents' being overweight or obese.

While healthy food options may be in short supply in some communities, those same communities often suffer no lack of unhealthy options. Mehta and Chang (2008) found a positive association between availability of fast-food restaurants and higher individual weight. A number of other researchers have found similar results (Chen, Florax, and Snyder, 2009; Morland, Diez Roux, and Wing, 2006). Researchers have also found that children who have a fast-food restaurant within a tenth of a mile of their school have a 5.2 percent greater chance of becoming obese (Currie, Della Vigna, Moretti, and Pathania, 2009). And many companies use aggressive marketing tactics to promote unhealthy food, often to the most vulnerable communities. For example, the average American child watches 10,000 food commercials a year on television, of which 95 percent advertise foods that are either sugar-packed or high in fat (Berg, 2004).

For these reasons, many experts, such as Powell, Ham, and Chaloupka (2010), endorse a comprehensive strategy that includes cheaper prices (subsidies for healthy foods), greater availability (greater access to supermarkets in underserved communities), and increases in the cost of fast foods (through taxation). Each of these approaches, however, brings with it economic and political considerations and consequences.

Anderson (2008, p. 605) argues for a "rights-based" approach to food systems (RBFS): "Localization and a community base can help to achieve both sustainability and RBFS as they contribute to awareness of the environment and social costs of current food system practices."

One key component of food justice is *food security*, which the World Bank defines as "access by all people at all times to enough food for an active and healthy life" (Anderson and Cook, 1999, p. 142). Pinstrup-Andersen (2009) notes that this term has evolved; originally it meant that a country had sufficient access to food to meet the nutritional requirements of its residents. The term now has expanded to include how accessible healthy food is to all sectors of the population (Lutz, Swisher, and Brennan, 2010). In some circles, the term encompasses an added dimension of *food preference*, to include foods that are considered more desirable from a social or cultural perspective.

According to Hamm and Bellows (2003, p. 37), a critical element of the food justice movement is the ability to promote *community food security*, which is defined as "a situation in which all community residents obtain a safe, culturally acceptable, nutritionally adequate diet through a sustainable food system that maximizes community self-reliance and social justice." This perspective, which emphasizes *community capacity enhancement* (the systematic identification of a community's assets and incorporation of those assets into interventions) through the creation of local food production and marketing, democratic decision making, and ecological sustainability (Levkoe, 2006), parallels many principles found in social work and justice-related movements. The lack of access to healthy foods as a social justice issue has started to attract the attention of scholars across disciplines (see, for example, Christopher, 2008; Morgan, 2009; Robertson, Brunner, and Sheiham, 2006; White, 2007). Renzaho and Mellow (2010) also stress the importance of grounding the concept of food security within a localized context to ensure that it captures a cultural perspective of how it is defined.

It should be noted that some critics offer other reasons for the dramatic increase in obesity and overweight. Philipson and Posner (2008), for example, advance the "neoclassical theory of obesity," which is apolitical and identifies technological changes as the primary reasons for obesity (cheaper food translates into more eating and less need for physical labor at work and home).

Environmental Justice

The origin of any social movement is difficult to pinpoint. Thus, only rarely can a social movement be traced to a particular moment in time or a specific individual or organization (Hawken, 2007). Nevertheless, an attempt to trace the origin is very important in order to better understand the circumstances that galvanized a community to act.

There is general agreement that the environmental justice movement originated in early attempts to account for illnesses resulting from exposure to toxins and pollutions, and eventually found its application to health risks such as obesity (Taylor et al., 2008). During its evolution, the environmental justice movement has expanded beyond health consequences to encompass social, economic, and political damages to groups and communities.

Walker and Bulkeley (2006) contend that environmental justice has its origins in the civil rights movement. Ash, Boyce, Chang, and Scharber (2010) more specifically trace the birth of this movement to the publication of *Toxic Wastes and Race in the United States* (Commission for Racial Justice) in 1987, which focuses on environmental disparities resulting from race and low income. The 1979 *Bean v. Southwestern Waste Management* case is considered the first legal suit to address environmental racism based on civil rights law (Bullard, 2005c). This case highlighted a local effort to establish a municipal landfill near an African American community in Houston, Texas. The case was successfully argued using civil rights laws that showed the potential impact of environmental racism on a community of color.

Initially, the term *environmental racism* referred specifically to the role of race in the environmental justice movement (Faber, 1998; Rhodes, 2003). Eventually, such terms as *environmental injustice, environmental justice activism*, and *environmental equity* emerged as a way of broadening the concept to involve other social factors such as class (Brodkin, 2009; Lester, Allen, and Hill, 2001; Sze, 2007), and in the process, deemphasized the highly charged concept of racism. *Environmental racism* seeks to capture the disproportionate effects of environmental pollution on communities of color. *Environmental justice*, in contrast, captures race along with socioeconomic class and other significant factors, since people of color tend to be segregated into low-income geographical settings (Sze, 2007).

The environmental justice movement has evolved tremendously since its conception and presents a prism through which to view the effects of structural factors, such as unequal protection from regulatory agencies, on health and obesity (Agyeman, 2005; Lee, 2002; Schlosberg, 2007; Sze, 2007). Morland and Wing (2007, p. 171) address how this movement has expanded: "The environmental justice movement brought racial and economic discrimination in waste disposal, polluting industries, access to amenities, and the impacts of transportation planning to the public's attention."

Taylor (2000) proposed an environmental justice paradigm emphasizing an injustice framework for understanding the relationship between people and their environment, which has increased awareness of environmental problems in which communities of color are disproportionately affected (Brulle and Pellow, 2006). Simultaneously, it has also been responsible for developing an all-encompassing definition of health to include physical, social, cultural, and spiritual factors, empowering residents to demand the right to reside in healthy, livable, and sustainable communities (Lee, 2002).

As environmental justice evolves, it affects multiple disciplines, broadening its framework to include an expansive list of socio-environmental concerns (Walker, 2009). Among these, scholars and activists are beginning to include disproportionate access to health-promoting community resources, such as parks and sidewalks, and subsequent health risks within marginalized communities, as environmental justice issues (Handy and Clifton, 2007; Taylor et al., 2006).

A natural extension of this is the concept of food justice. The concept of food security overlaps with that of environmental justice when climate changes or environmental practices severely affect food production and accessibility, leading to health and social consequences (Battisi and Naylor, 2009; Ebi, 2009).

Lutz et al. (2010, p. 2) sum up the dynamic:

> The evolution of community food security is a response to growing problems in many food systems in the world. Community food security addresses several key issues facing modern food systems, both on a local and global level. The concept of community food security is unique in its intention to examine the complex relationships between crucial characteristics and components of food systems. This holistic approach involves issues from community members' ability to obtain food, to the social welfare of the workers and participants in the food system. While some of the individual components of this view of food systems are still in the development stage, the overall idea of a "big picture" approach to food systems problem solving and management is a positive addition to food security efforts around the world.

Gottlieb and Fisher (1996) urged food and environmental justice groups to form coalitions because of the tremendous overlap between these two movements. Gottlieb (2009, p. 7) argues that both address "issues of health, globalization, worker rights and working conditions, disparities regarding access to environmental (or food) goods, land use and respect for the land, and, ultimately, how our production, transportation, distribution, and consumption systems are organized."

Winne (2009, p. 8) summarizes the growing merger of the food and environmental justice movements: "Hunger, supermarket abandonment of urban America, and a growing discontent with food and the environment emerged as separate but equal problems in the 1960s and gradually swelled to a tidal wave by the 1980s. Each to varying degrees had its own antecedents, champions, and constituencies. They chose different projects and solutions, mobilized their respective constituencies, and enjoined political figures to intervene as they saw fit."

The environmental impact of many food industry practices is also criticized. For example, 185 million barrels of oil—more than was spilled off the Gulf Coast by British Petroleum in 2010—is used to produce the 96 billion pounds of food that are discarded in the United States every year (Main, 2010).

An environmental perspective would also consider the massive amounts of animal waste produced by our food supply, and the health consequences that result when it enters our water and food systems (Weeks, 2007). The Environmental Protection Agency estimates that hog, chicken, and cattle waste has been responsible for polluting an estimated 35,000 miles of rivers in 22 states and contaminating groundwater in 17 states (Weeks, 2007).

Anderson (2008) discusses how "pesticide drift" merges issues of food activism, public health, and social justice. Pesticides affect the environment in both good and bad ways, and contact with pesticides has a deleterious effect on the health of agricultural workers. Furthermore, consumption of pesticides has profound effects on health. While such environmental issues are beyond the scope of this book, they are significant to those who study the interrelation of food and environmental justice.

Gottlieb (2009, p. 7) proposes an interesting way of conceptualizing both food and environmental justice as a means of bridging these two important movements: "One crucial way to expand the reach and breadth of the environmental justice movement and environmental justice action and research agendas would be to extend the environmental justice slogan that the environment is 'where we live, work, and play' to include 'where, what, and how we eat.' The linkages between environmental justice and food justice approaches can extend beyond traditional notions of environmental or food issues to address issues of health, globalization, worker rights and working conditions, disparities regarding access to environmental (or food) goods, land use and respect for the land, and, ultimately, how our production, transportation, distribution, and consumption systems are organized." The separation of these two movements, I and others would argue, is artificial (Sze and London, 2008).

Spatial Justice

Pirie (1983) is often credited with popularizing the concept of spatial justice back in the early 1980s (Dikec, 2001). The concept has started to gain popularity in academic circles that study the over-representation of social problems within distinct geographical areas, such as low-income urban communities of color. A spatial justice lens is not restricted to any particular geographical frame of reference, and is relevant in urban, suburban, exurban, and rural settings. However, it certainly enjoys tremendous popularity when applied to an urban context (Fainstein, 2010; Harvey, 2009).

Soja (2010) has constructed spatial justice as a theoretical concept, a method for conducting empirical analyses, and a viable strategy for creating social and political action. Spatial justice provides practitioners and academics with a geographical lens through which to better assess the equitable distribution of resources, services, and access, all three of which are key elements in understanding overweight and obesity among the nation's urban communities of color (Soja, 2010). Social work, however, has not embraced this perspective, even though our practice is contextualized and stresses the importance of the relationship between geographical setting and undervalued groups.

Geographical areas that experience the deleterious consequences associated with poverty, for example, share a distinct socioeconomic profile that highlights class, race, and ethnic characteristics (Hay, 1995; Holifield, 2001; Pearsall and Pierce, 2010). These areas ("inner-cities," "distressed areas," "barrios," "blighted communities," "ghettos") have a disproportionate number of residents with chronic diseases, ex-inmates, low-wage groups, female-headed households, undocumented newcomers, alcohol outlets, psychiatric facilities, toxic-waste dumps, diseases, substance abuse, fast-food restaurants, and other social problems (Fainstein, 2008, 2010; Harvey, 2009; Livingston, 2008). Such high concentrations, in turn, serve to marginalize the communities within the broader society, by creating an environment that fosters loss of hope and dignity.

Spatial justice raises often overlooked issues related to people rather than to systems and physical objects: walkable streets, access to healthy food, green space, toxic-waste sites, for example. Consider the finding that nationally, low-income zip codes have 30 percent more convenience stores than middle-income zip codes have. These convenience stores, in turn, are less likely to sell fresh fruits and vegetables than are supermarkets in middle-class neighborhoods (Treuhaft and Karpyn, 2011).

This encompassing perspective shows great promise for application in fields that specifically attempt to address the relationship between places, spaces, and social and health problems, such as overweight and obesity, in low-income/low-wealth urban communities of color. It takes on even greater relevance in better understanding urban communities, as noted by Brand (2007, p. 8): "While theories of justice often situate themselves directly within the space or time of the city, they do create a framework for understanding the production of injustice and conversely, the production of justice." Edwards (2010) utilizes spatial analysis techniques to study obesogenic environments in order to better understand the concentration of risks for obesity, such as availability of fast-food establishments, access to playgrounds and parks, and safety of streets for walking. Cooper and Page (2010) use GPS technology to obtain highly detailed spatial-related objective measures that can help explain obesity rates in certain communities. This approach facilitates a view of the severity of the problem in a way that lends itself to wide interpretation.

Spatial justice can complement the other perspectives often associated with overweight and obesity (Soja, 2010, p. 13): "Spatial justice is not a substitute or alternative to other forms of justice but rather represents a particular emphasis and interpretative perspective. I have also argued that foregrounding a critical spatial perspective and seeing the search for social justice as a struggle over geography increase the possibility of opening up new ways of thinking about the subject as well as enriching existing ideas and practices."

The Interaction Between Food, Environmental, and Spatial Justice

The subject of access to healthy food and opportunities for physical exercise for undervalued urban groups clearly transcends all three justice spheres. Nevertheless, each of these perspectives emphasizes a particular dimension that affects how we view the increase in overweight and obesity in this country, particularly among certain subgroups.

Schlosberg (2007, p. 5) both acknowledges the ambiguity associated with social justice movements and accepts it as part of the terrain of social justice–related work: "The argument here is that movements use a wide variety of conceptions of justice, and we can find arguments in these movements for distribution, recognition, participation, and capabilities. . . . For one, groups and movements often employ multiple conceptions of justice simultaneously, and accept the ambiguity that comes with such a hetero-geneous discourse."

The emphasis on food, environmental, or spatial justice dictates the lens through which we view the phenomenon of excessive weight and the language that we use to analyze and propose solutions. However, this does not mean that the other perspectives are lost. In essence, it becomes a question of foreground and background, depending on whether we em-phasize food, environmental, or spatial aspects. In addition, each of these perspectives has found its way into the health promotion field (Ash et al., 2010; Delgado and Zhou, 2008; Masuda, Poland, and Baxter, 2010).

Wekerle (2004) provides a conceptualization of food justice that lends itself well to environmental and spatial justice initiatives: (1) projects originating at the local level that serve as alternative practices, and set the stage for potential policy change initiatives, or those that are intra-community focused (Hess, 2009; Levkoe, 2006; Wallace, 2008); (2) inter-community state-focused efforts at altering policies (Born and Purcell, 2006; Gottlieb, 2009; Harrison, 2008); and (3) extra-community efforts that seek to develop networks at local and regional levels (Allen, 2008; Donald, Gertler, Gray, and Lobao, 2010; Gottlieb and Joshi, 2010).

As already noted, there can be a great deal of overlap among these three perspectives on social justice. For example, the lack of green space can be conceptualized from a variety of viewpoints depending upon which particular aspect we are emphasizing (Boone, Buckley, Grove, and Sister, 2009). Green space can encompass parks, trees, and gardens, for example. If the parks are unsafe because of criminal or gang activity, and not patrolled by police to the degree needed to make them safe, then a spatial justice perspective can be used. We can examine the number of crimes committed in this geographical area and compare it with that in other areas of the city.

If these parks are not usable because of pollution (near toxic waste sites, air pollution due to industries or car and bus fumes), or are simply uncared for (broken bottles, lack of adequate lighting, discarded needles, used as a dumping ground for cars, household appliances, etc.), then an environmental justice perspective can be used (Bullard, 2005a; Mohai and Saha, 2006).

A food justice perspective on available land, such as abandoned build-ing lots, or land available in public housing developments, suggests a third view. If the governmental authorities or private owners of such properties do not permit community gardens to be planted, food justice advocates can argue for such usage. Communities can quantify the extent of available use of land within their boundaries, using spatial justice for this form of analysis.

The reader may well prefer one social justice perspective over the others, depending on his or her experiences, knowledge base, and/or the organizational commitment of his or her place of employment (Hsu, Anen, and Quartz, 2008; Stanley, 2009). It is important to reiterate that no one perspective is more "worthy" than the others. Each viewpoint emphasizes a particular aspect of social justice, and fits with social work's mission to address oppression, and exercise participatory democratic principles in the process.

Each of these perspectives is employed throughout this book, as well as the overarching construct of social justice. Each will be used as a means of bringing together scholarly material from a variety of disciplines. Understanding these viewpoints helps create collaborations across disciplines, and minimizes misunderstandings about how best to address overweight and obesity in urban communities that are marginalized by society (Ewing, 2005).

Health Promotion and Social Justice

Health promotion brings together all of the key elements necessary to carry out action inspired by social justice (Wallerstein and Freudenberg, 1998). The health field, particularly public health, has begun to embrace social justice as a guiding paradigm. Ruge (2010), for example, advanced what is called the "health capability paradigm," which stresses the importance of access to the means for preventing premature death and morbidity.

Social action campaigns often represent a signature element of any social justice–focused health promotion intervention, and those focused on overweight and obesity are no exceptions. Munger (2003–2004), for example, proposes a campaign featuring Ronald McDonald as the next Joe Camel "poster child" to regulate fast-food advertisements targeting children. These symbolic figures play a critical role in mass advertising and are well known (Burns et al., 2009). Using these characters to convey a political message can help to galvanize public opinion in support of action.

Critics of fast food and other unhealthy foods call for a full-scale intervention similar to recent public health campaigns against smoking (which include higher taxes on tobacco, smoking bans in public places, restrictions on marketing cigarettes to children, and warning labels) (Brownell, 2010). These interventions seek not only to increase consumer awareness of the causes of overweight and obesity but also to mount campaigns to alter industry practices and implement governmental regulations to protect consumers.

Klein and Dietz (2010, p. 388) argue for the construction of a social justice campaign against childhood obesity similar to those efforts against smoking:

> Overcoming the childhood obesity epidemic will require changes on the scale of a social movement similar to the shift in attitudes and regulations toward smoking and tobacco. Tobacco control became a successful public health movement because of shifts in social norms and because cigarette companies came to be perceived by many as a common enemy. In contrast, obesity advocates have not identified a common threat or mobilized grass-roots change, nor have they identified strategies that resonate across diverse settings and constituencies. Framing obesity as a common threat can lead to consensus regarding the interventions needed to achieve healthier children and communities.

Freeman (2007) argues that the fast-food industry relies on a close relationship with government in order to continue its practices of targeting marginalized communities in the United States and other countries. This complicity needs to be tackled by activists. Freeman goes so far as to advocate that the Food and Drug Administration create a branch specifically dealing with the fast-food industry.

Food justice advocates have also supported legislation that requires restaurants to label the nutritional content of the foods they serve. "The modern food environment has prompted the call for menu labeling. Few Americans eat recommended amounts of produce and many over consume calorie-dense, nutrient-poor foods. Obesity is one consequence, but increased risk for diseases related to poor diet (e.g., heart disease, cancer, diabetes) is a concern for the entire population" (Pomeranz and Brownell, 2008, p. 1578).

By 2009, menu-labeling legislation had passed in 13 cities, counties, and states (those states being California, Maine, and Oregon), with New York City being the first major city to pass the law (Mantel, 2010). Advocates of menu labeling are quick to note that placing labels on menus will not by itself reduce excessive weight. However, it is part of a comprehensive effort to do so (Mantel, 2010). The restaurant industry, not surprisingly, has voiced strong opposition to these efforts by arguing that it is too costly, impractical, and finally, that it violates a restaurateur's right to free speech.

Evaluation Rewards and Challenges

Social workers who embrace a social justice paradigm face challenges when it comes to evaluating their efforts. One facilitator summarized the obvious challenges of evaluating community perspectives on obesity prevention (Whitacre, Burns, Liverman, and Parker, 2009, p. 27): "Despite the power of community experience, researchers and policy experts have found it difficult . . . to articulate the 'hows' and 'whys' of that experience and how it should inform and influence our work."

Kumanyika (2005) offers a word of warning about embracing an advocacy stance:

> In public health, because of our commitment to advocacy, there is always the danger of becoming a *believer*—becoming so convinced about the issues one is pursuing that it becomes difficult to consider new information objectively. Although a degree of subjectivity is inherent in all scientific inquiry, one who believes uncritically risks missing opportunities to progress based on new insights, or, worse, one may introduce bias into inquiry—selectively evaluating data or studying the question in a way that favors a certain answer.

This does not mean that social workers using a social justice paradigm cannot carry out "scientifically" sound evaluation. It does mean, however, that we must make explicit the values and principles guiding our evaluation efforts. All too often evaluation efforts emphasize the "scientific" values of methodology and analysis and leave values and principles implicit. Overweight- and obesity-related interventions must be explicit if the socioecological forces underlying excessive weight gain are to be understood and addressed.

Further, these rewards and challenges must be cast against a host of other challenges that the field is facing nationally and internationally. Aicken, Arai, and Roberts (2008, p. 1) sum up the state of the field regarding effectiveness of interventions:

Both internationally and in the UK, there is widespread concern about rising rates of overweight and obesity and the consequences of this for individuals, for population health and for the wider society. This concern is not yet matched by either a clear map of interventions provided for children and young people or a robust evidence base on the effectiveness of interventions. The potential range of such interventions is very wide, with sound evaluation facing both methodological and practical challenges.

Careful attention to evaluation design, as a result, has increased in importance as the field has started to acknowledge the complexities in addressing excessive weight within, and across, population groups.

The dissemination of results goes far toward inspiring other communities to duplicate, and innovate, by illustrating what is feasible and sharing the lessons learned. Community change efforts offer much promise in combating various industries and their lobbying efforts. However, the failure to critically evaluate these undertakings is a serious problem that must be successfully solved in order for consumer- and community-led initiatives to move forward (Brownell, 2007).

The Extent of the
National Obesity Crisis

These facts lead many to conclude that the time for concerted action to reduce levels of obesity and the deleterious effects of obesity is clearly upon us. In preparing for such action and in an attempt to enlist the participation and aid of broad sectors of society, many believe that labeling obesity a disease and having society accept this label is vital. However, is the label warranted? Prominent obesity experts have offered the opinion that it is indeed warranted, but equally prominent (although fewer) obesity experts have disagreed.
(ALLISON ET AL., 2008, P. 1116)

To put a face on the obesity crisis, we will examine how it has evolved and identify which groups in the United States are most at risk. Excessive weight can best be understood from historical, evolutionary, and contextual points of view; thus a social context is critical for developing an in-depth understanding of the issue.

Every effort will be made to make this discussion both informative from a statistical perspective and also "reader-friendly" in light of the vast amount of research on obesity that has been conducted over the past several years and that will not diminish in the foreseeable future (Wang and Kumanyika, 2007).

National Statistics

Any serious review of national statistics on overweight and obesity will quickly overwhelm all but the most knowledgeable experts on the subject. Although the topic has surely not suffered from lack of quantitative data, the paucity of data on obesity among significant subgroups is striking (Finkelstein and Zuckerman, 2008).

The trend toward greater and greater weight gain across all groups is undeniable. In 2007, the daily caloric intake of the average American was 400 calories higher than in 1985 and 600 calories higher than in 1970 (Whelan, Russell, and Sekhar, 2010). As noted earlier, a net increase of only 100 calories per day may result in a 10-pound weight gain for an average individual over the course of a year. These increases are particularly significant in low-income urban communities of color.

Wang and Beydoun's (2007) review of the literature found that among adults, obesity rates more than doubled (from 13 percent to 32 percent) between 1960 and 2004. In 2004, two-thirds of all adults were either overweight or obese, and 16 percent of all children and adolescents were overweight, with an additional 34 percent being at risk for being overweight. Annual prevalence increases ranged from 0.3 to 0.9 percent across all groups. After reviewing data for the past decade, Spruijt-Metz (2011) concluded that childhood and adolescent obesity is an epidemic in the United States and worldwide.

The impact can also be examined from state and regional perspectives. It has been recently estimated that 30 percent of the nation became obese from 2007 to 2009 (Grady, 2010). Nine states (Mississippi, Alabama, Tennessee, West Virginia, Louisiana, Kentucky, Oklahoma, Arkansas, and South Carolina) had populations that measured more than 30 percent obese during a three-year period (CalorieLab, 2010). Mississippi (34.4 percent) had the highest obesity rate of any state (Grady, 2010). In California, 60 percent of adults and 30 percent of youth are either overweight or obese (California Health Policy Forum, 2009). Northeastern and western states had the lowest adult obesity rates in the country (Levi, Vinter, St. Laurent, and Segal, 2010), and Colorado was the "leanest," with 18.9 percent of its population being classified as obese.

States and cities with high percentages of low-income people of color bear a disproportionate burden of this weight crisis, since weight gain is not evenly distributed across the entire population. Arizona does not appear among the top 10 heaviest states, for example, but in its Latino community, 33 percent are classified as obese (Innes, 2010).

Obesity Rates Among Various Subgroups

Recent attention to health disparities in marginalized communities of color in the United States has highlighted the challenges that these communities face (CDC, 2010a; Richardson and Norris, 2010), since they are disproportionately at risk for overweight and obesity, with the attendant deleterious health and economic consequences.

The health inequities in these communities, combined with their continued projected growth in population, have significantly increased the importance of the topic among public policy officials, academics, and practitioners. The subject of health care costs, however, invariably takes center stage and unfortunately pushes the subject of what causes illness and health disparities out of the spotlight.

Kumanyika (2001) provides a useful framework for better understanding the causes of excessive weight in communities of color by identifying issues in three aspects of the community's environment: (1) physical environment (lack of access to healthy foods and excessive access to unhealthy foods); (2) sociocultural environment (high-caloric traditional foods and unfavorable attitudes toward physical exercise); and (3) economic environment (lack of access to physical spaces/places due to lack of money and scarcity of safe and accessible green areas such as parks and playgrounds).

The interrelationship of environment, community, individuals, and families must be appreciated and understood in the case of people of color living in urban communities. This grounding, in turn, informs policy development, research, and interventions that are context- and group-specific and have relevance for all levels of social work practice.

Robert and Reither (2004) concluded that the determinants of obesity are multiple and multi-level, posing incredible challenges for the development of interventions, particularly those that are narrow in scope (which tend to be popular from a research standpoint). Social interventions are most effective when they are targeted to specific groups and subgroups, and are "place"-sensitive. A scattershot approach does not differentiate between subgroups, thereby limiting its effectiveness. It can also result in a sense of futility if progress is not made.

Many studies suggest the complex interplay among race, ethnicity, age, gender, and other factors in overweight and obesity. For example, Baum (2007) highlights the strong effects of race, ethnicity, and age on obesity. Zhang and Wang (2004, p. 1171), in a study of adults 18–60 years of age, found it necessary to examine the interplay of gender, age, and ethnicity in order to better understand obesity in communities of color: "Consistent with previous studies, we found remarkable ethnic differences in the relationship between SES [socioeconomic status] and obesity. Although the extant literature documented a higher prevalence of obesity among minorities than in whites, our results presented a lower socioeconomic inequality in obesity within minority groups. Our analyses suggested that gender, age, and ethnicity could be important factors on socioeconomic inequality in obesity."

The following sections examine obesity and overweight as related to five factors: race and ethnicity, age, gender, socioeconomic status, and urban environment. I have selected these categories because of their particular importance for those who advocate for social justice. Despite the significant overlap among these factors, it is possible to focus on the unique aspects of each category without losing sight of its interconnectedness with the others.

Race and Ethnicity

"Minority" status in this country brings with it a host of social, economic, political, and health consequences, of which excessive weight is but one example (Teran, Belkin, and Johnson, 2002). Although the problem of overweight and obesity occurs across virtually all sectors, certain other racial and ethnic groups have higher prevalence rates than do white, non-Latinos (Kumanyika, 2005).

Native Hawaiians/Pacific Islanders have by far the highest prevalence of obesity in the country; 63.5 percent of those 18 and older are obese, a rate that is 1.6 times that of white, non-Latinos (Office of Minority Health, 2011d). African Americans/blacks have the second-highest prevalence of obesity in the country (CDC, 2009); 33.2 percent of those 18 and older are obese, a rate that is 1.5 times higher than that of white, non-Latinos (Office of Minority Health, 2011a). The rate among Latinos, in comparison, was 1.2 times higher than among white, non-Latinos, with 31.7 percent classified as obese (CDC, 2009; Office of Minority Health, 2011c).

Asian Americans have a *lower* rate of obesity when compared to white, non-Latinos—three times lower—with 12.5 percent being obese (Office of Minority Health, 2011e). Native Hawaiians/Pacific Islanders were 3.7 times more likely to be obese when compared to the overall Asian population (Office of Minority Health, 2011d). Korean Americans had the lowest percentage, with 2.8 percent being obese. Finally, American Indian/Alaska Natives were 1.6 times more likely to be obese than were white, non-Latinos, and 34 percent of their population falls into the obese category (Office of Minority Health, 2011b).

Populations who are new to this country face special issues when it comes to obesity and weight. The concept of *dietary acculturation* explains how eating patterns and attitudes toward exercise may change as a result of adjustment to a new cultural environment (Satia-Abouta, 2003). Yeh, Viladrich, Bruning, and Roye (2008) argue that acculturation must not be viewed unilaterally and that a selective acculturation perspective better captures the complexity of the process. One recent study, for example, found that Asian newcomers to America may eat unhealthy American food because they want to fit into American society, even if the new dietary choices are counter to their cultural upbringing (Guendelman, Cheryan, and Monin, 2011).

The term *Hispanic paradox* has emerged to highlight how acculturation among Latino newcomers has translated into unhealthy lifestyles, including eating disorders (Chamorro and Flores-Ortiz, 2000; Hayes-Bautista, 2002). Latino newcomers are healthier than their USA-born counterparts upon entering the United States, even though they have lower incomes and less access to health care (Delgado, 2007). However, the longer they reside in the United States, the less healthy they become, even though their incomes rise and they gain increased access to health care (Lara, Gamboa, Kahramanian, Morales, and Bautista, 2005).

Levels of Latino acculturation have thus been identified as important considerations in intervention development (Bowie, Juon, Cho, and Rodriguez, 2007, p. 8): "Our finding that the percentage of Hispanics who are overweight or obese increases with acculturation also suggests that one approach to reducing rates of overweight and obesity and improving the overall health of Hispanics might be to encourage them to maintain their traditional dietary practices." Perez-Escamilla (2011) found evidence in the literature to support an association between acculturation level, and poor dietary quality and obesity. Similarly, Liou and Bauer's (2010) study of obesity perceptions among Chinese Americans highlighted the struggles of bridging the "old" culture and the "new" culture.

It is critically important to reiterate here that culture should not be used to blame the victim for being overweight (Kaufman and Karpati, 2007). It is possible to prevent obesity among racial and ethnic groups while concomitantly supporting healthy traditional diets and physical exercise that reinforce cultural identity and pride (Latino Coalition for a Healthy California, 2006).

Age

Age plays a prominent role in dictating the type and place of interventions to prevent, identify early, and treat overweight and obesity. We will address three age groups here: (1) children and youth (Field, 2007a; Mayer, 2009; Nanney, 2007; Stettler, 2007); (2) adults (Phelan, Butryn, and Wing, 2007); and (3) adults 65 and older (Morland and Filomena, 2008; Newman, 2009). Each of these age groups covers a significant period of the life span; however, in the interests of simplifying the discussion, each will be treated as a unit, for the most part.

CHILDREN AND YOUTH

It is appropriate to start with children and youth (Singh, Kogan, Van Dyck, and Siashpush, 2008). This age group has benefited from increased attention and, some would argue, alarm because of the long-range health implications for overweight and obese children (Whelan, Russell, and Sekhar, 2010). Adolescents who are overweight have a 70 percent chance of being overweight or obese as adults, and that likelihood increases to 80 percent if one or both parents are also obese (Surgeon General, 2007). It may be that children and youth who are surrounded by individuals (family, neighbors, and classmates) who are overweight or obese develop an inaccurate perception of what constitutes "normal" or "typical" weight (Maximova et al., 2008).

It is estimated that childhood obesity has increased by 300 percent in the past 25 years (Skelton, Cook, Auinger, Klein, and Barlow, 2009). In 2003–2004, 17.1 percent of all children and adolescents in the country were overweight (Ogden et al., 2006).

The picture is even grimmer for children and youth of color:

- Obese, low-income preschool children of color increased from 12.4 percent of all preschool children in 1998 to 14.5 percent in 2003 and 14.6 percent in 2008 (*Morbidity and Mortality Weekly Report,* 2009).
- Kimbro, Brooks-Gunn, and McLanahan (2007) found that African American and Latino 3-year-olds are at particular risk for being overweight and obese. Preschool children who are obese are at increased risk of entering adolescence and adulthood as obese, with profound social and health implications (*Morbidity and Mortality Weekly Report,* 2009).

- Not surprisingly, since diabetes is positively correlated with obesity, children in marginalized urban communities account for almost 50 percent of all new cases of type 2 diabetes (Whelan, Russell, and Sekhar, 2010).
- Children and youth of color have been particularly hard hit by this increase, and they are frequently underserved by this nation's health care system (Crothers, Kehle, Bray, and Theodore, 2009)
- Some experts contend that young children will likely "outgrow" this weight as they transition out of this age group. However, that may not be the case for some children of color, African American children for example (Lee et al., 2010).
- Delva, Johnston, and O'Malley (2007) note that youth of color, particularly males, were more likely to have a body mass index (BMI) at or above the 85th percentile, a measure that is inversely associated with eating breakfast, fresh vegetables and fruits, and regular exercise.
- Wang, Gortmaker, and Taveras (2010) found that the prevalence of "severe obesity" among youth in this country is increasing at a rapid rate, particularly among Latino boys and non-Latino black girls.

It is estimated that in general, four or five students in a typical classroom would be classified as obese. However, in a population of low-income youth of color, approximately half of all students in high school would be classified as obese (Koplan, Liverman, and Kraak, 2005; Schwimmer, 2005; Viner and Macfarlane, 2005). This percentage is expected to continue to increase if no substantive effort is made to stem the tide of excessive weight in this group.

ADULTS

The Centers for Disease Control and Prevention (CDC, 2011a) reported that one-third (33.8 percent) of all adults in the United States could be classified as obese in 2010. The number of American adults who were obese increased by 1.1 percent (2.4 million) between 2007 and 2009 (Yanovski and Yanovski, 2011). However, adults of color bear a disproportionate share of the problem with obesity (Calzada and Anderson-Worts, 2009; Osel-Assibey, Kyrou, Adi, Kumar, and Matyka, 2010).

African American adults had the highest rates of obesity (44.1 percent), followed by Mexican Americans (39.3 percent), all Latinos (37.9 percent), and white, non-Latinos (32.6 percent) (CDC, 2011b). Asian Americans as a whole, however, were three times less likely than white, non-Latinos to be obese, with 8.1 percent. For Asian American subgroups, Filipinos had the highest percentage (14.1 percent) and Korean Americans had the lowest (2.8 percent). However, these rates were almost twice those of their counterparts in Korea (Cho and Juon, 2006).

OLDER ADULTS

It has been estimated that 37 percent of those 65 and older were obese in 2010; if current trends continue, that figure will increase to 50 percent by 2030 (Sommers, 2009). Newman (2009) summarizes prevalence among older adults this way:

> By 2000, the prevalence of obesity in people 50 to 69 years of age had increased to 22.9%, and for those above 70 years of age to 15%, representing increases of 56% and 36% respectively, since 1991. . . . Although the prevalence of obesity in persons who are over 80 years of age is about one-half that of older adults between the ages of 50 and 59, the fact is that more than 15% of the older American population is obese. . . . Moreover, as the aging population increases in number, so too will the number of chronic illnesses, which often accompany aging, increase in our society.

Obese older adults also experience a lower health-related quality of life (HRQOL) than those who are either overweight or of typical weight (Groessl, Kaplan, Barrett-Connor, and Ganials, 2004). Reynolds, Saito, and Crimmons (2005) found the impact of obesity on active life expectancy in older adults (70 years and older) to be minimal, but they also found that obese older adults are more likely to become disabled. Zabelina, Erickson, Kolotkin, and Crosby (2009) found that excessive weight had both positive (less impairment of self-esteem and public distress), and negative (greater difficulty with physical function, sexual life, and work) consequences for older adults.

There is general agreement that prevalence rates for obesity increase with age, along with increases in high blood pressure, increased levels of LDL cholesterol and triglycerides, and increased onset of type 2 diabetes (Taylor, 2002). Maintaining a healthy level of physical activity also becomes more important as a strategy to offset the effects of a slowing metabolism. These factors, along with the importance of maintaining a healthy diet, necessitate development of comprehensive intervention strategies for older adults that are distinct from those aimed at youth (Delgado, 2009).

Gender

Women, particularly women of color, evidence higher levels of obesity than men. Prevalence of obesity among adult women is 35.5 percent, while among men it is 32.2 percent (Flegal, Carroll, Ogden, and Curtin, 2010). Women of color are particularly at risk for obesity, with 51 percent of African American/black women aged 20 years or older being obese, compared with 43 percent of Mexican Americans and 33 percent of white, non-Latinas (CDC, 2011c).

As briefly discussed earlier, societal values of thinness have put undue pressure on women. Women may encounter greater discrimination and be the subject of excessive marketing of "solutions" to overweight and obesity to a greater extent than their male counterparts. Bhattacharya and Bundorf (2009), for example, argue that a substantial portion of the lower wages among women who are obese can be attributed to labor market discrimination because of higher health insurance premiums.

Interventions that are gender-focused are increasingly common and reflect the growing awareness of how weight issues are manifested differently according to gender. Simen-Kapeu and Veugelers (2010), for example, argue for the need to have gender-specific interventions when addressing overweight and obesity in children, due to gender differences in physical activity and nutrition.

Researchers have concluded that body mass distribution varies by gender, and therefore age, obesity, and gender should be taken into account when working with anthropometric data sets, which are a collection of civilian and military surveys that cover a 50-year period (Chambers, Sukits, McCrory, and Cham, 2010). Borders, Rahrer, and Carderelli (2006) specifically highlight how low-income women of color, for example, have significantly increased odds of being overweight or obese, and should be targeted for specific interventions.

The bias against weight gain and excessive weight is far greater for women than men. It has been reported that even a modest weight gain can result in women's experiencing bias, and the figure for women is far less than that required for men to experience discrimination (Parker-Pope, 2008). The correlation between sexism and excessive weight further reinforces the need for a rights perspective and the importance of using social justice principles in the design of interventions that are sensitive to gender. The implications of this dual standard can be particularly deleterious for young girls who may struggle to achieve the "ideal" weight at any cost.

Socioeconomic Status (SES)

Research findings correlate socioeconomic class and overweight and obesity (Drewnowski and Specter, 2004; Whelan, Russell, and Sekhar, 2010). One study of neighborhood property values and zip codes found that for every additional $100,000 of median home price, the obesity rate declines by 2 percent (ScienceDaily, 2007). McLaren's (2007) extensive review of the literature on socioeconomic status and obesity found a strong positive association between low-income status and larger body size, particularly in industrialized nations.

Drewnowski (2004), in turn, argues that obesity in this country is primarily an economic issue, with the highest rates of obesity found in communities with the highest rates of poverty. Almost 25 percent (24.5) of adults (2007–2009) in the top quarter of household incomes ($50,000) were obese in the United States, and so were 35.3 percent of those with incomes of less than $15,000. Obesity prevalence decreases as income increases and also decreases as educational level increases, with 22.0 percent of those with a graduate school or technical school education being obese. However, 33.6 of those with less than a high school diploma were classified as obese (Levi, Winters, Laurent, and Segal, 2010).

These communities have limited access to healthy foods and physical space for exercise, increased access to fast-food restaurants, and are bombarded with an inordinate number of advertisements that encourage consumption of high-calorie foods.

Oliver (2006) argues that American adults are eating the equivalent of four meals per day and children almost the equivalent of five meals, meaning that our tendency to snack is a key factor in excessive weight gain. Availability of energy-dense snacks that provide a quick pick-me-up and then a crash, however, can be disproportionately high in low-income urban communities of color.

Lower socioeconomic groups have been found to consume fewer vegetables (Casagrande, Wang, Anderson, and Gary, 2007; Kant and Graubard, 2007), fruits (Casagrande et al., 2007; Kant and Graubard, 2007), whole grains (Harnack, Walters, and Jacobs, 2002), lean meats (Shimakawa et al., 1994), and low-fat milk (Johnson, Panely, and Wang, 2001; Shimakawa et al., 1994) than higher-income groups (Larson and Story, 2009). Lower socioeconomic groups have also been found to consume higher levels of sugar (Xie, Gilliland, Li, and Rockett, 2003) and sweetened drinks (Hendricks, Briefel, Novak, and Ziegler, 2006), making for a more energy-dense diet.

It is extremely arduous, however, to disentangle issues of class from those of race and ethnicity, given the history of slavery and racism in this country and the way these pernicious forces have forced major portions of communities of color into the lower socioeconomic classes and certain neighborhoods. Williams-Brown, Satcher, Alexander, Levine, and Gailer (2007), in a focused intervention on African American men who were upper-middle-class and affluent, found that they had much in common with their lower-income counterparts' health characteristics, raising the importance of race as a major influence on health when compared to SES. Mind you, the challenge of disentangling class, race, and ethnicity is not restricted to the problem of overweight and obesity; it also applies to other social problems. Interventions must not lose sight of social class and how it impinges on other demographic factors.

Urban Environment

The reader may question why "place" is listed along with the other factors in this discussion. I contend that place is a very important factor in shaping how groups encounter, and possibly address, the social forces that are operating to cause overweight or obesity (Walks, 2009; Wallace, 2008).

The spatial justice issues considered earlier help to frame the importance of geography (place and space) for better understanding overweight and obesity in urban communities, and in population subgroups within these communities.

Carr's (2007, p. 5) description of cities does a wonderful job of highlighting how urban context plays an influential role in residents' view of their immediate world:

Cities have often been places where different communities and cultures converge. This has generally taken the form of immigrants or migrants grappling with the culture of their new homeland and its indigenous people. However, alongside this natural tension of new populations living with older, established ones, there are also communities' interactions with the "culture" of the city itself. These large urban expanses are often places of extremes: severe poverty and excessive wealth, beautifully maintained open spaces and neglected streets with rundown housing, opportunities for innovation and enterprise and the potential for overwork and stress, the tolerance that stems from its diversity and the violence and crime that stems from fragmented and deprived communities. These familiar characteristics of life within a large city have a significant impact on the individuals living within them, including their ability and opportunities to take part in health promoting activities.

An ecological approach brings a contextual understanding that is not possible through a focus on individuals. "Urban sprawl," for example, has emerged as a causative factor in how this nation has increasingly gained weight. Time spent driving as opposed to walking has increased over the past several decades, lending credence to how lack of physical activity plays an influential role in weight gain (Frank, Andresen, and Schmid, 2004; Wen, Orr, Millett, and Rissel, 2006). However, there is considerable debate about whether urban sprawl is a significant factor in weight gain (Eid, Overman, Puga, and Turner, 2008; Ewing, Schmid, Killingsworth, Zlot, and Raudenbush, 2008; Lopez, 2004).

The promotion of "active travel" (walking and cycling) is an attempt to promote physical activity as an alternative to automobile transportation (Mackett, 2010). This form of travel, however, requires a conducive environment, with safe paths and roads, and free of crime.

Kumanyika and colleagues (2008), in an extensive review of the literature on population-based prevention of obesity, found that prevalence of obesity in rural areas (20.4 percent) was higher than in urban areas (17.8 percent) of the country. However, among children aged 6–9 living in urban areas, the rate was 26.1 percent, slightly higher than among those living in rural areas (22.8 percent) (Wang and Beydoun, 2007). Boardman, St. Onge, Rogers, and Denney (2005) found that urban neighborhoods characterized by a high proportion (25 percent or higher) of African American/black residents have a 13 percent increase in the odds of being obese when compared to other neighborhoods. Grow et al. (2010) found that neighborhoods characterized by multiple indicators of social disadvantage (social and economic context) experience increased risk for childhood obesity because of how racism and classism limit free mobility and possibilities for physical exercise.

Much of the attention on healthy food has focused on fresh fruits and vegetables. Hosler, Varadarajulu, Ronsani, Fredrick, and Fisher (2006), however, undertook a study of low-fat milk and high-fiber bread availability in rural and urban (Albany, New York) community stores and found that rural communities had a high probability of having low-fat milk (71 percent) and high-fiber bread (55 percent), when compared to urban stores (40 percent and 33 percent, respectively). Albany's people of color (80 percent), not unexpectedly, had limited access to low-fat milk and high-fiber bread, important items in a healthy-food diet.

Food Stamps and Obesity

The Supplemental Nutrition Assistance Program (SNAP), established in 1964 and commonly known as "food stamps" serves an estimated 38 million people, or one in 8 Americans, an increase from one in 50 in the 1970s (Vanderkam, 2010). The subject of overweight and obesity among food stamp recipients has generated attention, particularly since it is low-income groups that have experienced a disproportionate increase in overweight and obesity (Dinour, Bergen, and Yeh, 2007). The conclusions are mixed.

MkNelly (2009), in a review of the literature, found that food stamp recipients (children, adult men, and older adults), are not more likely to be overweight or obese. However, for adult women some evidence suggests that food stamps may increase the probability of obesity. Baum (2011), on the other hand, found that food stamps have significant positive effects on obesity. However, these effects were relatively small and had only a minor role in increasing obesity at the aggregate level.

One study of women who received food stamps, which controlled for socioeconomic status, found that they were more likely to be overweight when compared to their counterparts who were not receiving food stamps. In addition, they gained weight at a faster rate (*Science Daily*, 2009). Gibson (2003), too, found an association between food stamp participation, women, and obesity. Ver Ploeg, Mancino, and Lin (2006) found, however, that based upon 1999–2002 data, increases in BMI and obesity were more rapid among women who did not receive food stamps than among those who did.

Food stamps cannot be used to purchase tobacco or alcohol products. However, they can purchase soda and sweetened beverages. In New York State an effort is under way to ban the purchase of foods and beverages that are not nutritious (Farley and Daines, 2010). This proposed policy change is a direct response to the high rate of excessive weight in New York City.

Future Projections

Predicting the future is always a challenging task, and this is certainly the case when predicting future trends in overweight and obesity. Nevertheless, it is important to do so without taking a fatalistic viewpoint that there is nothing we can do. It does seem, however, as if all predictions agree that the prevalence of overweight and obesity, and their multifaceted consequences, will only increase in the near future. The debate, unfortunately, is more about the extent of the increase.

Some experts suggest that overweight and obesity rates will reach 75 percent of all adults by 2015 and 86.3 percent of this nation's adult population by 2030, if current trends continue (Wang and Beydoun, 2007; Wang, Beydoun, Liang, Caballero, and Kumanyika, 2008). However, the projected increases are even more dramatic for African American women (96.9 percent) and Mexican American men (91.1 percent). Other countries have not escaped these dire predictions either. The United Kingdom, for example, expects a 50 percent obesity rate by 2050 (Alvanides, Townshend, and Lake, 2010).

Communities of color are projected to continue dramatic increases in weight gain and obesity over the next 40 years, making the topic one of continuing importance among this group, particularly in urban centers of the nation.

Is the nation getting "fatter"? Yes. Is overweight and obesity a national crisis? Yes, particularly if we focus on subgroups within urban communities of color. Is there national outrage about this? Unfortunately, I believe that the answer is no. That is one of the primary reasons why this book was written.

The demographic factors highlighted here represent some of the most widely acknowledged variables on the subject of overweight and obesity. Other factors, not discussed here, include religious affiliation (Krukowski, Lueders, Prewitt, Williams, and Smith, 2010), the incarcerated, the homeless, individuals with physical or emotional disabilities (Hellerstein et al., 2007), and transgendered or bisexual people. These additional factors have generally escaped the attention of scholars, although practitioners can no doubt see their influence on food consumption and exercise. Breaking down generalized populations into subgroups of marginalized people further reinforces the importance of excessive weight interventions being subgroup-specific.

Health, Economic, and Social
Consequences of Obesity

One measure frequently used to quantify the health effect of obesity is premature mortality. Estimates of the number of obesity-related deaths vary widely, ranging from approximately 112,000 ... to 365,000 per year. ... Despite ongoing controversy over the exact number of associated deaths, obesity is clearly associated with increased mortality.
(COLDITZ AND STEIN, 2007, P. 74)

Being overweight or obese carries multifaceted consequences, both obvious and hidden, for individuals, families, communities, and society. These conditions are important not only because they influence our physical appearance in a society that worships "thinness" but also because of the effects of excessive weight on our quality of life. Obesity actually goes far beyond being considered a public health condition (Crosnoe, 2007). The costs and consequences of excessive weight have a profound impact on all spheres of daily life.

Although consequences have usually been framed from a health perspective, other consequences of overweight and obesity exist that have generally been overlooked. These further consequences, however, manifest a range of severity levels depending upon a host of factors such as socioeconomic class, age, neighborhood characteristics, race, and ethnicity (Berg, 2004; Lobstein, Baur, and Uauy, 2004; McLaren, 2007). Our task here is to describe a multifaceted foundation from which to appreciate the magnitude of these additional costs to individuals, families, communities, and the nation, and to examine the implications of such costs for the social work profession.

Muennig, Lubetkin, Jia, and Franks (2006) found that the consequences of overweight and obesity can be measured through lost quality-of-life years, which, simply defined, means the loss of the ability to enjoy life's possibilities and activities. (The saying "It is not the number of years in a life but the quality of life in those years" sums up what is meant by "quality-adjusted life years.") In Muennig et al.'s study, overweight men and women lost 270,000 and 1.8 million quality-adjusted life years, respectively, compared to their normal-weight counterparts. Obese men and women lost 1.9 million and 3.4 million quality-adjusted life years, respectively.

More specifically, a consideration of three dimensions can help us to capture a multifaceted view of the consequences of overweight and obesity: (1) health costs, (2) financial costs, and (3) social costs. These categories overlap to some extent, but each warrants focused attention, which can be accomplished without losing sight of the myriad interrelationships in play here.

Health Costs

The physical health consequences of overweight and obesity often get the most attention in the popular and scientific literature (Wolin and Petrelli, 2009). It is estimated that 300,000 deaths every year are the result of obesity (Flegal, Williamson, Pamuk, and Rosenberg, 2004). Colditz and Stein (2007), along with many others, have confirmed the connection between increased morbidity and mortality and excessive weight. Moreover, many researchers suggest that we may be underestimating the true physical and economic costs because the range of illnesses that have been directly attributed to overweight and obesity has been defined too narrowly.

A general appreciation of how health is influenced by excessive weight will help to clarify the discussion. Being overweight or obese triggers many specific health consequences. One estimate lists at least 30 obesity-related diseases and finds that obesity affects almost all organ systems in the human body (Ludwig and Pollack, 2009). Diseases and conditions such as cardiovascular disease, asthma, gallstones, various forms of cancer, diabetes mellitus, hypertension, hyperlipidemia, osteoarthritis, musculoskeletal problems, non-alcoholic fatty liver disease, and sleep apnea are often closely correlated with weight (Anandacoomarasamy, Caterson, Sambrook, Fransen, and March, 2008; Harrington and Elliott, 2009; Liburd, 2010b, c; McKinnon, 2010).

Among these associated diseases, it could be argued that diabetes has received the greatest attention (Liburd, 2010b, c). An estimated 6.3 million people in this country live with undiagnosed diabetes (ChallengeDiabetes .Com, 2009). Being overweight or obese is considered a major risk factor for diabetes in communities of color, as compared to white, non-Latino communities (Office of Minority Health, 2007).

African Americans face the greatest threat from diabetes and are twice as likely to be diagnosed as white, non-Latinos; the highest incidence of diabetes occurs among those in the 65–75 age group. Twelve percent of African American women over 20 years of age have diabetes, as do 8.5 percent of men in the same age group. African Americans are also more likely to suffer from complications from the disease (Office of Minority Health, 2007, p. 1): "Diabetic retinopathy, an eye disease, is 40 to 50 percent more common in African Americans than Whites. Kidney failure (end-stage renal disease or ESRD) is about 4 times more common in African Americans with diabetes than in Whites with diabetes. Amputations of lower extremities (legs and feet) are also more common in African Americans with diabetes."

Other groups of color also face health challenges related to diabetes. In 2002, two million Latino adults (approximately 8.2 percent of that population) were diagnosed with diabetes. The prevalence of diabetes among older Latinos is also severe, with about 25 to 30 percent over the age of 50 having the disease. It is important to note, however, that it is estimated that almost one-third of Latinos with diabetes go undiagnosed. They are 1.5 times as likely to have diabetes as white, non-Latinos, and in 2001 it was estimated that the death rate from diabetes among Latinos was 40 percent higher than that among white, non-Latinos. Mexican American adults, in particular, are 1.9 times more likely to be diagnosed with diabetes than are white, non-Latinos (Office of Minority Health, 2010b). Christiansen (2008) notes that a variety of factors contribute to higher rates of diabetes among Latinos and African Americans, particularly factors related to diets.

Diabetes is the fifth leading cause of death among the Asian and Pacific Islander community (Office of Minority Health, 2007). It is estimated that 11 percent of this group has been diagnosed with diabetes (Office of Minority Health, 2010a). Native Hawaiians, Japanese, and Filipino adults living in Hawaii are twice as likely to be diagnosed with diabetes as white, non Latino residents. Native Hawaiians/Pacific Islanders are three times as likely to be diagnosed with diabetes as white, non-Latinos and 20.6 percent of their adult population (age 18 or older) has this disease (Office of Minority Health, 2010c).

Finally, American Indians and Alaska Natives are two times as likely to be diagnosed with diabetes as white, non-Latinos (Office of Minority Health, 2007, p. 1): "As of 2003, 14.5 percent of the American Indian and Alaska Natives served by the Indian Health Service had been diagnosed with diabetes. The likelihood of having diabetes is higher in older age groups, with about 20 percent of American Indians and Alaska Natives between 45 and 64 having diabetes, and about 23 percent of American Indians and Alaska Natives over age 64 having diabetes."

Obesity and type 2 diabetes (a chronic disease involving high levels of glucose in the blood, requiring medication to move blood sugar into cells) have been shown to be closely associated with socioeconomic status, with the highest rates found among those with the lowest formal education and income, and in communities with high concentrations of residents who have these characteristics. Further, obesity, type 2 diabetes, and communities of color are highly associated. Drewnowski (2009, p. S39) brings a socioecological assessment to the conditions that give rise to high rates of obesity and type 2 diabetes: "Given economic constraints, especially among lower-income groups, not all consumers have the same degree of choice when it comes to purchasing healthful fresh produce, fruit, lean meats, and fish. For many, the choice was removed long ago by economic and employment policies. There are sound economic reasons why poverty and obesity are so closely linked, and this could affect future obesity-prevention strategies."

It is even more troubling to note that children are now experiencing many of the same obesity-related diseases, such as type 2 diabetes and high blood pressure, as adults. However, in children the time interval between the onset of obesity and the emergence of obesity-related health problems is considerably shorter. One estimate suggests that obesity-related diseases take 10 years to emerge in adults, but only three to five years in children (*Biotech Business Week*, 2010). Children who are overweight or obese and have type 2 diabetes are also at increased risk of needing coronary bypass surgery before they reach the age of 30 (Brownell and Horgen, 2006).

Diabetes is only one of the diseases associated with overweight and obesity; unfortunately, these conditions can often lead to a host of illnesses.

Excessive weight brings an increased incidence of heart disease, thereby increasing the likelihood of heart attacks, congestive heart failure, sudden cardiac death, angina, and abnormal heart rhythm.

People of color have a higher prevalence of hypertension (high blood pressure), a major risk factor for cardiovascular disease, than do white, non-Latinos (Redman, Baer, and Hicks, 2011). Excessive weight plays a critical role in hypertension, and hypertension, in turn, contributes to racial/ethnic disparities in morbidity and mortality. African American/ blacks and Mexican Americans had a 40 percent greater likelihood of developing hypertension than did white, non-Latinos, after adjustment for socio-demographic and clinical characteristics.

Strokes, too, are a major health risk related to obesity and communities of color (Trimbal and Morgenstern, 2008). Approximately 780,000 people in the country have either a new or a recurrent stroke every year. However, African American men are twice as likely as white, non-Latino males to have a first stroke (Covington et al., 2010). Almost 4 percent (3.9 percent) of all African Americans aged 18 and older suffered a stroke in 2009 (Office of Minority Health, 2010d). They were also 70 percent more likely to die from a stroke than were white, non-Latinos.

Latinos, surprisingly, have a lower risk of stroke than their white, non-Latino adult counterparts (Office of Minority Health, 2010g). Two percent of all Latinos over the age of 18 have suffered a stroke. Women have a higher likelihood (2.3 percent) than men (1.6 percent). Latinos are less likely to die from a stroke, and they have lower rates of hypertension and high cholesterol than do white, non-Latino adults.

Native American/Alaskan Native adults as a group are 60 percent more likely to have a stroke than are their white adult counterparts (3.6 percent), and their women are twice as likely (4.3 percent) to have a stroke as white, non-Latinas (Office of Minority Health, 2010e). Asian Americans are half as likely (1.3 percent) as white, non-Latinos (2.6 percent) to suffer a stroke (Office of Minority Health, 2010f). No data are available on cerebrovascular diseases and Native Hawaiians/Pacific Islanders as this book goes to press (Office of Minority Health, 2010h).

Financial Costs

The measurement of financial costs of diseases and illnesses is always subject to debate, and the costs (both current and projected) associated with excessive weight can be part of that debate. Estimating the financial cost of obesity is contingent upon how obesity is defined (McCormick, 2007). Colditz and Stein (2007) concluded that the escalating prevalence of overweight and obesity is matched by the challenges in quantifying the costs of this national health problem.

The average American may not associate overweight and obesity with financial costs; insurance companies and governmental sources are more concerned with these measures. Yet the financial costs of being overweight or obese have profound implications for individuals, families, employers, and the government. Cawley (2007, p. 612) offers a very sobering assessment of the state of affairs with regard to the cost-effectiveness of prevention: "It is clear that the best strategy for the long run is to conduct the necessary cost-effectiveness research so that policymakers, educators, and public health officials can find and implement the antiobesity interventions that yield the greatest gains for society. However, the best strategy for the short run—while such cost effectiveness data are still lacking—is less clear."

According to the American Diabetes Association, the estimated cost of diabetes in the United States in 2007 was $174 billion, of which $116 billion was attributed to medical costs and $58 billion to lost productivity (Petersen, 2007). It is estimated that in 2008 the nation spent $83 billion on hospital-related costs, or $10,940 per hospital stay, which averaged one day longer (5.3 days) than hospital stays for patients who were not diabetic (Raloff, 2010).

In 1998 it was estimated that obesity-related costs accounted for $78.5 billion, with half being paid by Medicare and Medicaid (Finkelstein, Trogdon, Cohen, and Dietz, 2009). One early 2000 estimate for hospital costs for children who were obese put the figure at $127 million a year, up from $35 million (a 300 percent increase from 1981) (Elias, 2002). The same study found that overweight Americans incurred $93 billion a year in medical costs (Hellmich, 2003). In 2008, the estimate increased to $147 billion, of which $7 billion was spent on Medicare prescription drugs (Finkelstein et al., 2009). Obesity is estimated to increase the costs for typical, non-obese employees by an average of $150 a year, based on 1998 dollars, or $25.6 billion in extra premium costs (Engelhard, Garson, and Dorn, 2009).

Another estimate suggests that health care costs resulting from overweight and obesity will double every decade—and will rise to between $860.7 and $956.9 billion by 2030, representing 16–18 percent of the total health care costs in the country (Wang, Beydoun, Liang, Caballero, and Kumanyika, 2008). Fiegar (2005) estimates that 3.7 percent of all medical expenditures result from those who are overweight and 5.3 percent from those who are obese. A 2009 estimate had obesity-related costs at between 5 percent and 7 percent of all annual health care expenditures (Ludwig and Pollack, 2009).

The California Health Policy Forum (2009) estimated that total health care and productivity costs related to overweight and obesity in California accounted for $21 billion in 2006. An investment of $10 per resident per year in effective community-based interventions would translate into a savings of $12 billion from California's obesity-related health costs within five years. The importance of prevention and early intervention speaks for itself.

However, the financial costs must take into consideration a range of socio-demographic factors in order to arrive at a more realistic estimate. Yang and Hall (2007) found that older adult males (65 years and older) spent 6–13 percent more in lifetime health care costs than men of "normal" weight. Older adult women (63 years and older), in turn, spent 11–17 percent more than their counterparts of "normal" weight. The financial costs associated with obesity in pregnancy, too, need to be examined from both immediate and long-term perspectives (Rowlands, Graves, de Jersey, McIntyre, and Callaway, 2010).

Such discussions of direct costs, which tend to garner the most national attention, do not include the many indirect costs associated with overweight and obesity, such as restrictions in daily activities, premature death, production losses, early retirement, and disability pensions. These aspects are rarely part of the national discourse, but they are of great importance to social work and to the quality of life of those who are either overweight or obese.

For example, Durden, House, Ben-Joseph, and Chu (2008) found that adjusted direct and indirect costs were higher for workers with elevated BMI than for those of normal weight. The indirect costs have been assigned to six categories: (1) absenteeism, (2) disability, (3) premature mortality, (4) presenteeism (reduced work productivity), (5) workers' compensation, and (6) total indirect costs (Trogdon, Finkelstein, Hylands, Dellea, and Kamal-Bahl, 2008). One 2010 estimate that incorporated a variety of costs not normally taken into account—such as spending extra money on gasoline by relying on a car rather than walking or utilizing public transportation—arrived at an annual cost for obesity (sick days, lost productivity, and other non-medical expenses) of $4,879 for women and $2,646 for men (Neergaard, 2010).

Reduced work productivity is a good example of an indirect cost of overweight and obesity. An extensive review of the literature found a positive relationship between obesity and sick leave (Neovius, Johannson, Kark, and Neovius, 2009). One study estimated the increased medical expenditures and absenteeism associated with obesity at an estimated dollar figure of $285,000 per year for firms with 1,000 employees, or $285 per employee (Finkelstein, Fiebelkorn, and Wang, 2005). Individuals who are obese have increased workers' compensation claims due to injuries on the job in high-risk occupations (Ostbye, Dement and Krause, 2007). Employees who are obese miss an estimated 20 days of work per year (Engelhard, Garson, and Dorn, 2009).

Another financial factor is the tremendous amount of money spent by Americans looking to reduce weight or avoid gaining more of it. The diet industry is a multibillion-dollar enterprise, and the money that consumers spend on diets comes out of increasingly smaller discretionary budgets (Derenne and Beresin, 2006; Solovay, 2000). It is estimated that 55 percent of Americans, or approximately 160 million individuals, are on a diet of some type at any given time (Stewart and Korol, 2010). Hill (2004) contends that this industry has grown proportionally to the growth of the overweight and obesity problem.

In 2003, diet medicines were estimated to cost consumers, primarily women, $40–$100 billion a year (Cummings, 2003). The emergence of expensive and risky surgical procedures (such as gastric bypass) to address obesity reflects the desperation of some individuals to solve the problem of their weight concerns when diet and exercise do not work (Greenblatt, 2003).

The popularity of "health foods," and products that are advertised as "organic," "natural," and "whole" foods has also grown tremendously. This industry earned $37.3 billion in 2008, up from $28.2 billion in 2005 (Singer, 2011). There are concerns that such foods may not be any healthier than common brands, which raises the possibility of involving federal regulators (such as the Federal Trade Commission) to investigate the claims made in advertising these products. Finkelstein and Zuckerman (2008) use the term "ObesEconomy" to capture the wide reach of economic incentives and consequences of excessive weight (including the diet industry, the health and fitness industry, and the food sector).

It is important to state here that effective prevention efforts can reduce the costs related to obesity. However, as noted by Van Baal et al. (2008), this decrease may be offset by an increase in costs resulting from the onset of unrelated diseases that will be experienced during an increased life span that extends into older age. Consequently, improved health care will result in a decrease in excessive weight-related costs, but this is not a "cure" for increased health expenditures. Promises of "savings" may prove hollow when the unanticipated costs are not taken into account.

Social Costs

The health and economic consequences of overweight and obesity can be measured by various calculations. The social costs are much more difficult to measure, but they can certainly be significant for those who are overweight or obese. Some studies suggest that individuals face low self-esteem and mental health consequences from living with these conditions over a sustained period of time; others contest that assertion (Brownell, 2007). The mental health aspects of overweight and obesity are quite complex (Strine et al., 2008). Here we can only summarize some of the key findings from the research related to obesity, discrimination, self-esteem, and depression.

Ironically, "fatness" was once celebrated (Oliver, 2006, p. 63):

> After all, to be fat in isolation simply means having plenty of stored calories, but to be fat in a society of limited resources means that one has the political power to have command over a finite food supply. In this way, fatness has connotations that go beyond its pure biological function—it is also a visible display of one's authority and prestige. Like wearing flashy jewelry or expensive clothes today, body fat historically has been a marker, not just of wealth, but of social dominance.

In modern mainstream American society, and many Western societies, excessive weight no longer conjures up images of privilege and social dominance. Instead, it is associated with the opposite. Individuals who are severely overweight or obese face discrimination in virtually all aspects of life in this country (Solovay, 2000). Yet there are virtually no legal or social sanctions against discrimination based upon weight (Andreyeva,

Puhl, and Brownell, 2008). This omission means that those who are overweight or obese are even more disenfranchised because they do not share the same legal recourse that other groups have if their rights are violated (Pomeranz, 2008, p. S96): "Unlike African Americans and gays, obese individuals have generally not been the subject [of] discriminatory laws aimed at depriving them of their civil rights. Nonetheless, obese persons have suffered from social and institutionalized biases that need to be addressed in their own unique form. As such, antidiscrimination legislation may be necessary."

It is estimated that the prevalence of weight discrimination in the United States is comparable to that of race discrimination, particularly among women (Puhl and Heuer, 2009). Solovay (2000) outlined how overtly and covertly discriminated against overweight and obese individuals are in this society, and why they face such a difficult road in getting their situation recognized. Puhl and Heuer (2010) go so far as to argue that the stigma of obesity threatens health, causes health disparities, and compromises obesity intervention efforts.

Gee, Ro, Garvin, and Takeuchi (2008) found that racial discrimination was positively associated with increased BMI and obesity among Asian Americans, a finding that reinforces why social justice is an appropriate lens through which to better understand overweight and obesity in communities of color.

Extreme care must be taken to avoid increasing the stigma associated with obesity in general, and among children in particular (McLean et al., 2009). The consequences of obesity are particularly important among school-aged children because of the many physical and emotional developments that are associated with this age period (Haines and Neumark-Sztainer, 2006; Johnson, Cohen, Kasen, and Brook, 2002). Low self-esteem caused by body image dissatisfaction can have numerous unintended consequences across the life span. One study of overweight El Salvadoran youth, for example, found that they had higher levels of body size dissatisfaction, lower peer esteem, and unsuccessful attempts at losing weight (Mirza, Davis, and Yanovski, 2005). Contradictorily, Wardle and Cooke's (2005) review of the literature on childhood obesity found that despite moderate levels of dissatisfaction with body weight, relatively few children who are obese were depressed or had low-self-esteem.

Wyatt, Winters, and Dubbert (2006) note that with an increase in weight-related illnesses, there is also a significant incidence of depression.

De Wil et al. (2010) found a significant positive association between depression and obesity for females, and a non-significant association for males.

Thus the jury is still out on the mental health consequences of excessive weight. However, there is no denying that individuals who are overweight or obese must contend with many daily trials and tribulations, in addition to the discrimination that they encounter that can result in serious emotional issues. Although the evidence is not conclusive, the mental health repercussions take on added significance for those who are already discriminated against because of their color and their income.

The conditions of overweight and obesity have consequences that go far beyond the issue of "attractiveness." When combined with a host of other high-risk factors, excess weight increases the likelihood of morbidity and mortality. These consequences take a disproportionate toll on those who have a low income, live in urban centers, and are people of color. These "risk factors" translate into health disparities for those who are either overweight or obese, with dramatic implications for their families and their communities.

The consequences associated with overweight and obesity can be measured in a variety of ways. Unfortunately, consequences related to money and financial costs seem to take center stage in most discussions. However, these consequences can also have an impact on lifestyles, lead to lost potential, and have tremendous social consequences, all of which need to be examined and given more attention in the media.

Lack of Access to Healthy Foods

For millions of Americans—especially people living in low-income communities of color—finding a fresh apple is not so easy. Full-service grocery stores, farmers' markets, and other vendors that sell fresh fruits, vegetables, and other healthy foods cannot be found in their neighborhoods. What can be found, often in great abundance, are convenience stores and fast food restaurants that mainly sell cheap, high-fat, high-sugar, processed foods and offer few healthy options.
(TREUHAFT AND KARPYN, 2011, P. 7)

Treuhaft and Karpyn's statement sums up poignantly the lack of healthy foods in low-income urban communities of color and the over-representation of fast-food establishments targeting this customer base.

Johnson (2010, p. 165) captures the challenges of finding a fresh apple in urban communities of color in this country:

Imagine you are standing on Martin Luther King, Jr. Boulevard in a neighborhood composed of over 90% African Americans. You visit all of the fast food restaurants and discover that over 80% of the menu items are fried in lard and are high in sodium. The healthy food items, such as fresh fruit, are in very short supply. You then spend the day listening to a local African American radio station and observe that the commercials for the fast food establishments in the area advertise only fatty food items on the menu. The next day you visit a majority Caucasian neighborhood in the suburbs and discover the opposite—over 80% of the menu items are healthy food choices and all of the radio commercials advertise the sale of healthy food items. No one would then be surprised to learn that residents in the African American neighborhood are substantially more overweight and unhealthy than residents in the Caucasian neighborhood.

Everything about the subject of food is political, and the sooner we understand and embrace this perspective, the sooner we can arrive at equitable solutions to the problem of overweight and obesity: "We recognized that food is at once a very personal and intimate thing while at the same time part of a political system that can at times unite and at others further stratify society. Few other systems touch people's daily lives in such an intimate way and offer an opportunity to exert larger political influence" (Ona, as quoted in Corburn, 2009, p. 114).

It is not possible to view overweight and obesity from a socioecological perspective without an in-depth discussion of the instrumental role that the food industry has played, and continues to play, in this crisis. Thus it is necessary to examine the impact of fast-food restaurants and convenience stores; the food industry as a source of food and employment; the impact of "big box" stores such as Wal-Mart; the role of schools; issues of food security and food justice; and the role of the government.

Fast-Food Restaurants and Convenience Stores

Developing an assessment of food outlets in urban communities can be challenging because of the varied places where food can be purchased. Project CAFÉ (2007) identified 10 sources for the purchase of food in a low-income Los Angeles neighborhood: (1) supermarkets, (2) convenience/liquor/corner stores, (3) convenience stores with gas, (4) specialty food stores (fish markets, meat markets, bakeries), (5) full-service restaurants, (6) fast-food restaurants, (7) carryout eating places (non-chain fast food), (8) carryout specialty items (coffee, donuts, smoothies, ice cream), (9) bars and taverns, and (10) mobile food trucks. I would add one other possible source: food sold out of a private residence (Delgado, 2011). Consequently, any comprehensive assessment of food access must encompass a variety of settings. First, however, we will focus on two particular sources of unhealthy foods: fast-food restaurants (called quick-service restaurants, QSR, in industry terms). Another popular type of chain is fast casual restaurants (FCR), such as Chipotle, Cosi, and Panera Bread, which offer the convenience of fast food but with the ambience of casual dining. We will also discuss the selections available at convenience stores. As noted earlier, low-income urban communities have a preponderance of such establishments (Booth, Pinkston, and Poston, 2005).

Why are chain restaurants like these of particular concern? An examination of the nutritional values at the top five fast-food restaurants (Burger King, Kentucky Fried Chicken, McDonald's, Taco Bell, and Wendy's) and the top five family restaurants (Applebee's, Denny's, Outback Steakhouse, Red Lobster, and Pizza Hut) found that their meals typically exceed the recommended levels of fat and calories (Brownell and Horgen, 2006).

The Cancer Project (2008) undertook a more targeted review, which assessed popular items at five of the nation's most popular fast-food restaurants: (1) Burger King (Breakfast Sausage Biscuit); (2) Jack in the Box (Junior Bacon Cheeseburger); (3) McDonald's (McDouble); (4) Taco Bell (Cheesy Double Beef Burrito); and (5) Wendy's (Junior Bacon Cheeseburger). The study found that these meals, not surprisingly, were high in fat, saturated fat, calories, sodium, and cholesterol, which have been strongly associated with increased cancer risk, overweight, and obesity. Items at many other chain establishments such as Applebee's (New England fish and chips, 1,910 calories), Chili's (Big Mouth Bites, 1,930), and Chipotle (chicken burrito, 1,750), do not fare much better (Mantel, 2010). Ruby Tuesday's Ultimate Colossal Burger with all the trimmings weighs 2.5 pounds and has 1,677 calories!

Striffler (2005, p. 31) points out that many of these chains have become progressively unhealthier over the past few decades: "Worse yet, the healthier alternatives seemed to get less healthy during the 1990s. McDonald's grilled chicken sandwich put on 140 extra calories from a thick layer of mayo, while its Grilled Chicken Deluxe started out with three grams of fat but now has a whopping twenty grams of fat. But even this hefty sandwich is surpassed by Burger King's BK Broiler, with its astonishing twenty-nine grams of fat."

Recent trends on the part of fast-food restaurants and supermarkets to offer healthy alternatives (through options such as salads) have much promise, and reflect how the industry can be responsive to market demands. However, it is still important to emphasize that these businesses are rarely found in low-income communities, thereby limiting their potential impact on many of the marginalized groups addressed here. Further, even if healthy options are available, cost considerations may effectively make them unaffordable for low-income households.

Fast-food restaurants are readily available to consumers with minimal time to eat and limited budgets, and are open to accommodate all three meals and late-night snacks, too. In 2011, for example, McDonald's increased the number of restaurants open 24 hours per day (Chase, 2011).

This convenience both reflects and encourages a recent transformation in American eating habits. In the 1960s, 75 percent of all meals were eaten at home; today the majority of meals are prepared or eaten outside of the home (Schlosser, 1988a, 1988b). In 1970, 25 percent of all household funds spent on food were spent on away-from-home eating. In 1995, that figure had grown to 40 percent; in 1999, it represented 47.5 percent; and in 2010, it was estimated to have reached 53 percent (Dave, An, Jeffery, and Ahluwalia, 2009). It is estimated that more than 40 percent of all American adults eat a meal at a restaurant on any given day (Brownell and Horgen, 2006). In the early 2000s, there were an estimated 858,000 restaurants in the United States and the average household spent $2,116 per year on food outside of the home (Brownell and Horgen, 2006). Back in 1998, Schlosser commented on how fast-food spending dominated the American budget: "Americans now spend more money on fast food than they do on higher education, personal computers, software or new cars. They spend more on fast food than on movies, books, magazines, newspapers, videos and recorded music—combined" (Schlosser, 1998b).

According to the National Restaurant Association, fast-food sales were expected to reach $168 billion in 2011. Eating out has become a new American tradition (Inagmi, Cohen, Brown, and Asch, 2009, p. 683): "In 2003, 41 percent of family food budgets were spent eating out. Fast food sales, which comprised more than 41 percent of restaurant sales, have increased from $16.1 billion in 1975 to $123.9 billion in 2003."

A focus on one particular city (Los Angeles) can help to illustrate how completely fast-food establishments and convenience stores dominate the food landscapes of many urban low-income communities (Project CAFÉ, 2007). In 2003, the Los Angeles County Department of Health Services called obesity rates "alarming" (L.A. Health, 2003), yet they have continued to rise. Between 1997 and 2005, obesity rates increased for all major groups in Los Angeles: Latinos (from 17.1 percent to 28.7 percent); African Americans (22.2 percent to 27.7 percent); young adults aged 18–29 (13.1 percent to 16.6 percent); adults 65 or older (13.1 percent to 16.6 percent); males (13.5 percent to 21.8 percent); and females (16.7 percent to 20.0 percent) (L.A. Health Trends, 2006). An estimated one-third of all youths under the age of 18 are classified as overweight, which is higher than the county average. Thus Los Angeles is a useful geographical location from which to study the linkage between food sources and obesity.

Kipke and colleagues (2007) studied the food establishments within walking distance of a school in East Los Angeles, a predominantly Latino community. They found 190 food establishments in the neighborhood, of which 93 (45 percent) were fast-food restaurants and 120 (63 percent) were within walking distance of the school. Of the 62 grocery stores, 18 percent sold fresh foods, but only 18 percent of those were within walking distance of the school. Limited public transportation options make community residents more dependent upon buying locally. Further, researchers found that there were only five parks in this community, with a total area of only 37.28 acres, or 0.543 acres per 1,000 residents; the lack of park space severely limited options for physical exercise.

Azuma, Gilliland, Vallianatos, and Gottlieb's (2010) study of three Los Angeles communities came to similar conclusions: "Of the 1,273 food establishments mapped in the 3 neighborhoods, 1,023 met the criteria of 'retail food outlet.' The most common types of retail food outlets were fast-food restaurants (30%) and convenience/liquor/corner stores (22%). Supermarkets made up less than 2% of the total. Convenience/liquor/ corner stores offered fewer than half of the selected healthful foods and sold healthful foods at higher prices than did supermarkets." Access to food in these communities is not the problem; access to healthy food, however, is (Ghirardelli, Quinn, and Foerster, 2010).

Los Angeles is by no means the only city that provides an illustration of these issues. In a study of New York City's Harlem neighborhood, Galvez et al. (2009) found convenience stores on 55 percent of the surveyed blocks, and fast-food restaurants on 41 percent. They also found a positive association between increased body size and availability of these establishments. Bodor, Rice, Farley, Swalm, and Rose (2010), too, in a New Orleans study, found that easy geographical access to fast-food restaurants and convenience stores was positively associated with weight and BMI gain.

In a study of three low-income communities in Nashville, Tennessee, Freedman (2009) found that convenience stores and non-chain grocery stores far outnumbered all other types of stores. There were a total of 33 stores within a one-mile radius of the three communities, of which 21 were convenience stores, 2 were supermarkets, and 10 were local markets. Not surprisingly, tobacco and alcohol products were consistently more prevalent than all varieties of fresh fruits, vegetables, or milk (Freedman, 2009, p. 393): "Disparities in local food environments represent one stone in the sea of influences affecting the health of the public, and the ripple effect provided by these differences may contribute to health inequalities."

Morland and Everson (2009), too, found a positive association between prevalence of obesity in communities where there were fewer supermarkets and more small grocery stores or fast-food restaurants. The authors concluded that types of food stores and restaurants influence food choices, with diet-related health consequences.

Bustillos, Sharkey, Anding, and McIntosh (2009), however, note that healthy food may be present in nontraditional types of food stores. Their study, based on two rural Texas counties, found that canned fruits and vegetables, whole-wheat bread, and whole-grain cereal were available in dollar stores and other establishments not noted specifically for selling food.

Overall, though, there is a strong association between inequities in food availability and race/ethnicity (Galvez et al., 2009). Kwate, Yau, Loh, and Williams (2008, p. 32) contend that in the case of African Americans, racism and segregation have combined to create this unhealthy situation:

Despite evidence that Black neighborhoods are disproportionately exposed to fast food, few explanations have been advanced to illuminate explanatory mechanisms . . . [as to why] race-based residential segregation is a fundamental cause of fast food density in Black neighborhoods. Segregation's effects on population and economic characteristics, physical infrastructure, and social processes work in tandem to increase the likelihood that Black neighborhoods in urban environments will bear a disproportionate burden of fast food restaurants.

So, how can we address this dilemma? Some local communities have confronted the proliferation of fast-food restaurants head-on. In early 2011, for example, the Los Angeles City Council passed an ordinance banning the establishment of new fast-food restaurants in a section of the city that is already saturated with such establishments (Medina, 2011). Gold (as quoted in Severson, 2008, p. A18) likened fast-food chains to "jellyfish in the ocean, with too many in one area, nothing else can thrive." In 2008 the city council passed a measure to encourage new grocery stores and restaurants with table service to open in this community as a means of introducing healthy options. Strum and Cohen (2009), however, argue that the fast-food-restaurant ban in South Los Angeles has not had the impact it sought to achieve in reducing excessive obesity rates, and they propose, instead, menu calorie labeling as a strategy that could potentially have a greater impact on overweight and obesity.

In 2010 San Francisco passed a law to remove toys from all fast-food meals that did not meet certain nutritional standards (fewer than 600 calories and fewer than 640 milligrams of sodium).

Other efforts are more global. An initiative by the Department of Agriculture offers a promising shift in policy (U.S. Department of Agriculture, 2010, p. 95):

> In order to reduce the obesity epidemic, actions must be taken to improve the food environment. Policy (local, state, and national) and private-sector efforts must be made to increase the availability of nutrient-dense foods for all Americans, especially for low-income Americans, through greater access to grocery stores, produce trucks, and farmers' markets, and greater financial incentives to purchase and prepare healthy foods. The restaurant and food industries are encouraged to offer foods in appropriate portion sizes that are low in calories, added sugars, and solid fat. Local zoning policies should be considered to reduce fast food restaurant placement near schools.

Similarly, the CDC (Khan et al., 2009, pp. 5–12) identified six strategies for promoting access to affordable healthy food and beverages. Communities should: (1) increase availability of healthier food and beverage choices in public service venues; (2) improve availability of affordable healthier food and beverage choices in public service venues; (3) improve geographic availability of supermarkets in underserved areas; (4) provide incentives to food retailers to locate in and/or offer healthier food and beverage choices in underserved areas; (5) improve availability of mechanisms for purchasing foods from farms; and (6) provide incentives for the production, distribution, and procurement of foods from local farms.

Another alternative to the fast-food movement is the "slow food" movement, which had its origins in a protest in Rome, Italy, to the opening of the first McDonald's in that city in 1987. The movement now has adherents in more than 140 countries, with a goal of promoting local cooking traditions, farming without pollution, and preserving endangered foods (Glazer, 2007). The mantra "good, clean, and fair" captures the central social, economic, and political goals of this movement, and why it is considered relevant to discussions of overweight and obesity in this and other countries.

The Food Industry as Employer

It would be simplistic to view the food industry as just a *supplier* of food. It is also a major employer, and that fact makes any sustainable effort at activism much more complicated. It was estimated that in 2003, one in seven jobs in the labor market was in franchise-related employment, representing more than $506 billion in private-sector payroll (Dant, 2008).

The fast-food industry has a long tradition of offering jobs featuring low pay, minimal benefits, and high employee turnover rates; in fact the term *McJob* has become synonymous with low-wage jobs and minimal career advancement. Fast food is one of the few business sectors that have positions available in this current dismal economy, particularly for applicants with little formal education or limited English-language skills. In mid-2011, for example, McDonald's announced a major hiring campaign seeking to add 50,000 new positions. Thus, any suggestion of regulation within the food industry is typically met with a concern that such a move will cost jobs, reduce tax income, and discourage business development.

Immigrants, in particular, make up a significant portion of the fast-food labor base. The number of immigrants employed in this sector was estimated at 1.8 million in 2010 (MSNBC.com, 2011). In 2009 the industry was estimated to have 25 percent of its workforce designated as "immigrant," with almost half (12 percent) of that group being undocumented.

Talwar (2002, p. 193) provides a chilling account of how newcomers have been absorbed into the fast-food industry as both customers and employees, and details the long-range social, economic, and political implications of this trend in the urban communities of color where newcomers settle. These establishments represent the initial point of entry into the labor force for countless people of color.

> We need to be attentive to the ways in which more and more immigrants are being absorbed into the corporate consumer world, whether they are flipping burgers at McDonald's, serving cappuccino at Starbucks, or taking movie tickets at Sony Theaters. And as these institutions become more numerous in immigrant neighborhoods—places thought to be immune to corporate growth—we need to be increasingly critical of the theories that isolate "ethnic economies," no matter whether fast food restaurants and corporate franchises are inextricably linked to ethnic economies or are their ultimate successor.

In 2010 a highly nationalized campaign targeted undocumented workers and raids by Immigration and Custom Enforcement (ICE). Chipotle Mexican Grill, whose motto is "Food with Integrity," was the target of one such campaign.

What are these jobs like? Greenfield (2011) describes the factory-like atmosphere in fast-food kitchens:

> Go into the kitchen of a Taco Bell today, and you'll find a strong counterargument to any notion that the U.S. has lost its manufacturing edge. Every Taco Bell, McDonald's, Wendy's, and Burger King is a little factory, with a manager who oversees three dozen workers, devises schedules and shifts, keeps track of inventory and the supply chain, supervises an assembly line churning out a quality-controlled, high-volume product, and takes in revenue of $1 million to $3 million a year, all with customers who show up at the front end of the factory at all hours of the day to buy the product.

Royle's (2010) study of employment practices of McDonald's and other U.S.-owned multinational fast-food corporations from the 1970s to the present documents how minimal employee progress has been achieved in that time period. Kanagui-Munoz, Garriott, Flores, Cho, and Groves (2011) found significant barriers in career advancement for Latino fast-food workers. In essence, these are entry-level and, with some exceptions, dead-end jobs.

Allen and Sachs (2007, p. 1) provide a nuanced perspective on the role of women in food provision: "Women perform the majority of food-related work, but they control few resources and hold little decision-making power in the food industry and food policy . . . although women bear responsibility for nourishing others, they often do not adequately nourish themselves." This gendered perspective on the food industry has generally been overlooked in the scholarly literature on food justice, which tends to be gender-neutral.

The Consolidation of the Food Industry

Global and national developments have led to the consolidation of the food industry, a point of concern to food justice activists because of the concentration of economic and political power it represents.

Brownell and Horgen (2006) highlight four of the major food corporations in the United States and list the various brands owned by each at the time of the inquiry; the results illustrate why the food industry wields such power:

(1) Kraft, which is owned by Philip Morris. Brands owned by Kraft include Baker's Chocolate, Breakstone, Breyer's, Country Time, DiGiorno, Good Seasons, Jell-O, Kool-Aid, Louis Rich, Maxwell House, Nabisco, Oscar Mayer, Philadelphia Cream Cheese, Post cereals, Stove Top, Toblerone, Tombstone Pizza.

(2) General Mills. Brands owned include Betty Crocker, Big G cereals, Bisquick, Colombo, Gold Medal, Green Giant, Häagen-Dazs, Jeno's, Lloyd's Barbecue, Nature Valley, Old El Paso, Pillsbury, Pop Secret, Progresso, Yoplait.

(3) PepsiCo. Brands owned include Aquafina, Aunt Jemima, Cracker Jack, Dole Juice Drinks, Gatorade, Frito-Lay, FruitWorks, Mountain Dew, Pepsi, Quaker, Rice-a-Roni, SoBe, Tropicana.

(4) ConAgra. Brands owned include Act II, Armour, Banquet, Brown 'n' Serve, Bumblebee, Butterball, Chef Boyardee, Chun King, Country Pride, Crunch 'n' Munch, Healthy Choice, Hebrew National, Hunt's, Knott's Berry Farm, La Choy, Libby's, Marie Callender's, Munch, Orville Redenbacher's, Peter Pan, Van Camp's, Wolfgang Puck's.

Food sources and suppliers are undergoing similar consolidation, further increasing the power of this industry. The meatpacking industry, for example, typifies this concentration of power, with four firms controlling 59 percent of the market in 2002, up from 19 percent in 1977 (United Food and Commercial Workers Union, 2010a). The four top companies involved in slaughtering hogs increased their market share from 36 percent in 1980 to 80 percent in 2007.

Food industry representatives would argue that these efforts to concentrate and consolidate have resulted in economies of scale, increased efficiency, and reduced food costs, ultimately benefiting the consumer. Nevertheless, critics contend that the food industry has failed to feed the hungry, produce healthy foods, or provide safe foods. It has also negatively affected workers in these industries, and consumers of their products (United Food and Commercial Workers Union, 2010b, p. 1):

Without a doubt, consolidation and concentration in the agricultural economy has caused decreasing incomes for farmers, ranchers, workers and the rural communities that depend on agriculture. Our rural communities, our food supply and the fate of a major portion of the American economy depend on us fixing this problem. However, we can't solve this dilemma unless we are willing to look at the whole picture of the American food chain—from the farm to the grocery store shelf.

Large retailers such as Wal-Mart enter into this discussion because of the influence they wield. Wal-Mart's share of U.S. grocery stores has increased more than 400 percent since 1978, and has more retail grocery sales than the next three largest competitors (Kroger, Safeway, and Supervalu) combined (United Food and Commercial Workers Union, 2010 a,b). This economic and political influence translates into Wal-Mart's controlling more than a 30 percent share in 44 percent of this country's major grocery markets. More specifically, it has more than a 50 percent share in 29 of those markets.

Four key questions must guide any analysis of the increasing consolidation of the food industry nationally and internationally (United Food and Commercial Workers Union, 2010a, p. 3): "It must be asked how did the distribution of the grocery store dollar get so skewed? What facilitated this shift? What impact has this shift had on workers and farmers? And what has this shift meant to rural agribusiness and rural economics?" The answers to these questions lay the foundation for why a social justice lens is needed, and why a social activism stance is required to offset the political influence of this sector.

Schools and the Food Industry

Children and youth face formidable obstacles in accessing healthy foods because their options are severely limited during the time they spend in school. Unfortunately, the choices available through many school lunches and snack machines have served only to introduce, or even reinforce, unhealthy diets (Nestle, 2007).

Schools have been an important target of the food industry for the selling of unhealthy snacks and beverages. Consider the consumption of sugared beverages. Sugary drinks account for almost 17 percent of an average adolescent's calorie intake in a day (Farley and Daines, 2010). They are called "liquid candy" because they have almost no nutritional value.

Yet they are ubiquitous; one study showed that sugary sodas could be purchased in 60 percent of all the nation's middle and high schools (Greenblatt, 2003).

In 2011 the mayor of Boston made national headlines by banning the sale and marketing of sugary drinks on city property. This response builds upon an earlier effort in 2004 when the Boston public schools banned sugary soft drinks from vending machines. Such bans are an expensive decision for schools. The banning of sodas by the Los Angeles Unified School District in 2004, for example, essentially resulted in $40 million lost revenues over a 10-year period since the money that the beverage industry paid to sell their product in schools was no longer available (Greenblatt, 2003).

In response, the National Soft Drink Association argues a variation of the personal responsibility argument (Greenblatt, 2003, p. 8): "It's the opinion of our industry that we should let parents decide what their children are eating and drinking in school. . . . It's that simple. I don't think any state or local government is better at making decisions for children than parents are." Dillard (2008) provides a scathing critique of the U.S. Department of Agriculture's school lunch program. Its policy of buying hundreds of millions of pounds of excess pork, milk, beef, and other forms of high-fat meat and dairy products has supported industry prices and concomitantly "dumped" these unhealthy foods onto students. Fortunately, efforts at redressing this injustice have begun. In 2010, the passage of the Healthy, Hunger-Free Kids Act extended and expanded school nutrition programs and also mandated that the U.S. Department of Agriculture increase its standards for school meals and nutrition by 2013. In 2009, 20 states and the District of Columbia had nutritional standards that exceeded U.S. Department of Agriculture requirements, an increase from six states in 2005 (Levi et al., 2010).

Other developments are also promising. Twenty-eight states and D.C. have established nutritional standards for foods sold in schools (such as through vending machines, school stores, and bake sales), representing an increase from six states in 2005. Efforts to introduce healthy snacks in school vending machines have increased, although getting students to select these snacks over less-nutritious choices is an uphill battle (Hu, 2011).

Twenty states officially require body mass index (BMI) screening for children and adolescents, representing an increase from four states in 2005 (Levi et al., 2010).

Other research projects promise intriguing results. In 2011, a San Antonio elementary school was selected to participate in an innovative program involving the analysis of uneaten lunch food, funded by the Department of Agriculture. The research will be used to calculate how many calories students eat and to identify what food is left uneaten (Associated Press, 2011). Parents who agree to participate in this program will receive regular reports on their children's eating patterns.

Farm-to-school programs have proliferated, from an estimated 10 in 1998 to more than 1,100 in 2007 (Joshi, Azuma, and Feenstra, 2008). These programs establish links to facilitate the purchase of fresh fruits and vegetables and delivery to schoolchildren, and often serve as a countermeasure in communities where fresh fruits and vegetables either are not available or are in limited supply. Farm-to-school produce costs are reduced by eliminating commercial establishments and their price markups. However, this movement is still in its infancy, since only 7 percent of the nation's students attend schools that offer such a program (Robert Wood Johnson Foundation, 2010).

School systems can address overweight and obesity among students through community-based collaborative efforts, such as those undertaken in Philadelphia's public schools (Moss, 2011). The U.S. Department of Agriculture has made changes to federally subsidized school meals (33 million lunches and 9 million breakfasts a day) that took effect in September 2012. The Philadelphia school system has banned soda, sweet snacks, and high-caloric fruit drinks from the schools and made an effort to have corner stores stock healthier foods. By early 2011, 507 of an estimated 2,500 stores had signed on to do so.

The importance of physical activities in schools must also be emphasized as a means of preventing overweight and obesity. The CDC identified four effective strategies to encourage physical activity among children and youth. Communities should (1) require physical education in schools, (2) increase the amount of physical activity in school PE programs, (3) increase opportunities for extracurricular activities, and (4) reduce screen time in public service venues. These four strategies can be used in various combinations to maximize positive weight-related outcomes.

Schools wield a tremendous influence in the lives of their students, families of students, and the community. Lessons learned at school can go beyond academics to include lifestyle choices, such as eating healthy foods and getting proper physical exercise. There is no reason that schools cannot be part of community efforts to address overweight and obesity, setting an example by bringing in healthier foods, expelling unhealthy foods, and providing opportunities for lifelong physical exercise.

Food Justice and the Food Industry

The emergence of "civic agriculture" represents one new perspective on food security that can have a great impact on the food industry. Proponents of civic agriculture endorse and support locally based agriculture and food production as an effort to counter the prevailing trends toward global agro-business (Lyson, 2004). The benefits of civic agriculture go far beyond offering community members easy access to healthy foods. They also encompass small-business development and increased social and human capital development. It is important to note that the globalization of the food industry is not restricted to processed foods. Counter-seasonal fresh produce, tropical products, and organic foods, too, are becoming an increasing part of the agro-food industry (Reynolds, 2004).

Food justice enters this narrative when some dimension of food accessibility is skewed in favor of or against a particular segment of the population. The issues of supply and accessibility make the concept of food security applicable globally, nationally, and locally for analyzing and describing various aspects of food justice. The San Francisco Bayview Hunters Point community, which will be discussed in detail in chapter 10, undertook an initiative, led by youth, in response to a lack of access to quality food. The partnerships that developed provide an example of how a food justice response relates to food security (Vasquez, Lanza, Hennessey-Lavery, Halpin, and Minkler, 2007).

The scientific merits of increasing consumption of healthy foods must be supported by a proven strategy for encouraging local businesses to sell these products. Numerous creative efforts for introducing healthy foods into low-income urban communities are under way or have been proposed. These initiatives must continue and be buttressed by government efforts to regulate the food industry, a goal that no doubt will encounter stiff opposition, given the economic power of the industry.

Limits to Places and Spaces
for Physical Exercise

Starved for parks and opportunities for urban recreation, and fed up with "No Soccer Allowed" signs, Latino voices are pushing for the transformation of the Los Angeles River from a vast concrete wasteland that winds through miles of Latino neighborhoods, to a ribbon of green space and parks that invite families and healthy activities.
(G. R. FLORES, 2008, P. 370)

The condition of overweight or obesity results from a complex interaction of individual and environmental factors. G. R. Flores's (2008) description of a Latino community in Los Angeles and its fight to positively alter the physical environment illustrates the struggles that low-income urban communities of color encounter in an effort to create safe and accessible spaces within their neighborhoods. The physical environment can be a force for either fostering or hindering activities that support health in low-income urban communities of color.

A social justice perspective provides a lens through which we can better understand the relationship between physical environments and health. Equity access and facility provision, for example, can be evaluated from a social justice standpoint (Jones and Panter, 2010). Lee and Cubbin (2009) advocate using a social justice lens to better understand disparities in physical activity, with particular attention to neighborhood characteristics (socioeconomic status, quality of housing, safety, access to quality health care, education, and occupational opportunities), and the impact of racial discrimination experienced in communities of color.

Policies and community/neighborhood infrastructure play a significant role in the prevalence of overweight and obesity (Macintyre, Ellaway, and Cummins, 2002; Sallis and Glanz, 2009). The lack of exercise due to an inability or unwillingness to engage in physical types of activities, too, must be considered in the development of interventions (Meyer, 2008). Availability and accessibility are especially important in urban communities, where safe places for physical exercise may be lacking (Jones and Panter, 2010; Pearce and Day, 2010).

The Built Environment

In 2006 the Federal Collaboration on Health Disparities Research identified the built environment as a key contributor to health disparities. The built environment usually encompasses urban design, land use, and transportation systems. Srinivasan, Liam, O'Fallon, and Dearry (2003, p. 1446) advance a more detailed and comprehensive definition:

> The built environment includes our homes, schools, workplaces, parks/ recreation areas, business areas and roads. It extends overhead in the form of electric transmission lines, underground in the form of waste disposal sites and subway trains, and across the country in the form of highways. The built environment encompasses all buildings, spaces and products that are created or modified by people. It impacts indoor and outdoor physical environments (e.g., climatic conditions and indoor/ outdoor air quality), as well as social environments (e.g., civic participation, community capacity and investment) and subsequently our health and quality of life.

The *built environment* is an umbrella term that brings together multiple fields of practice into an analysis of how the environment affects individual factors and choices.

Although there is a close relationship between the built environment and physical activity, research on the idea has been fragmented across different fields, resulting in lack of communication and collaboration (Day, Boarnet, Alfonzo, and Forsyth, 2006). Further, a focus on the built environment represents a significantly new development in research, away from social-cognitive theories and approaches (Van Lenthe and Brug, 2010).

There is an increasing trend in the field of public health to associate a variety of health issues and the built environment (Frumkin, 2002)

All geographical areas must contend with unanticipated negative consequences of a built environment. Cities, in particular, are subject to the forces unleashed by poorly conceptualized and constructed environments, with a particular impact on low-income communities. The interactions between built environments and social environments significantly alter the landscapes in which residents can engage in physical activities (Grow and Saelens, 2010). Lovasi, Hutson, Guerra, and Neckerman (2010), for example, illustrate how the built environment shapes obesity prevalence in "disadvantaged" urban population groups, and note the importance of creating environments that support physical activities.

Social scientists and public health researchers have begun to examine the impact of the built environment on other public health concerns, such as asthma (Brisbon, Plumb, Brawer, and Paxman, 2005) and depression (Kim, 2008). Cahill and Suarez-Balcazar (2009, p. 113) describe an appropriate built environment for children: "Every child in the United States should have the right to grow up in a safe, healthy, and supportive environment that affords them the opportunity to have a nutritious diet and healthy, active lives." Perdue, Stone, and Gostin (2003), in turn, promote the use of a legal framework for holding the built environment more accountable for health-related consequences, bringing a much-needed and overlooked role for public health advocates in the design of cities and suburbs.

The built environment takes on added significance for urban communities of color (McAlexander, Banda, McAlexander, and Lee, 2009, p. 705): "Community leaders must consider the association between the built environment and obesity in low SES areas when passing and/or enforcing public policies (e.g., increasing police surveillance, sidewalk and park maintenance) in order to treat and prevent obesity in this highly vulnerable population."

Macdonald (2007, p. 24) undertakes a systematic analysis of urban streets and identifies numerous ways that these environments waste space that could be productively utilized to increase quality of life for urban residents, including more space for physical activities: "For instance, streets can and should have a health function. Large numbers of Americans, especially children, suffer from obesity. . . . The linear nature of streets makes them ideal for walking, jogging and biking, and their distributed nature makes them readily available for everyone. Many people, however, will only use streets for exercise if they are attractive, comfortable and safe."

G. R. Flores (2008, p. 370) describes how a Los Angeles Latino neighborhood was positively transformed in the interest of increasing physical exercise for its residents through a relatively minor change in its built environment: "Nearby in Boyle Heights, Latino residents got a cracked sidewalk around a cemetery transformed into a 1.5 mile rubberized jogging path. Use increased from 200 to 1000 people a day walking, running, and socializing."

Cahill (2010) traces the environmental impact of transportation policy and how it has dramatically altered decision making among citizens, with profound consequences for the health of residents. Wilks (2010) examines the use of a child-friendly-cities (built environment and policies) framework to identify places for active citizenship by children and young people that result in healthy states of being. These spaces and places in a community increase social capital while concomitantly providing an opportunity to exercise.

Obesogenic Environment

An *obesogenic environment* is defined as "the sum of influences that the surroundings, opportunities, or conditions of life have on promoting obesity in individuals or populations" (Swinburn, Egger, and Raza, 1999, p. 564). The concept of the obesogenic environment extends beyond that of the built environment, emphasizing aspects such as street safety, walkable pathways, and public transportation. It also illustrates how the field of overweight and obesity has expanded beyond a focus on individual factors to one that takes into account cultural, social, and environmental forces (Lake and Midgley, 2010; Lake and Townshend, 2006; Lake, Townshend, and Alvanides, 2010).

Ball, Crawford, Timperio, and Salmon (2010) draw on the construct of the built environment and introduce the concept of the food environment (food availability, accessibility, and affordability) to capture how eating behaviors are affected by physical, sociocultural, and policy factors. This perspective, however, is relatively new in the field of obesity studies and opens the door for the introduction of social justice values and principles into the analysis of the problem, and the construction of place-based interventions (Alvanides, Townshend, and Lake, 2010).

The Importance of Physical Spaces in an Urban Context

Urban areas require a specialized discussion, particularly when examining excessive weight among low-income communities of color, which, incidentally, are heavily concentrated in cities. The evidence and knowledge regarding the relationship between population density and weight are mixed (Robertson-Wilson and Giles-Corti, 2010). However, we do know that street connectivity, housing design and structure, and modes of transportation all intersect in a unique configuration in cities, with profound implications for excessive weight gain.

Frank and Engelke (2001) were early proponents of examining the impact of the built environment upon urban quality of life, as manifested through health, safety, and social welfare. It is also important, however, to think about how various sectors of a community view the built environment. Krenichi (2006), for example, focused her research on women's physical activity in an urban park (in Brooklyn, New York) and the importance of attributes such as accessible rest rooms, freedom to wear comfortable clothes, hills, trails, a continuous loop, and safety to encourage utilization.

Rundle and colleagues (2007) advocate for mixed land utilization through more productive use of vacant or under-used land, and the reclaiming of *brownfields* (abandoned land that previously served industrialized or commercial purposes), which are often over-represented in older urban communities with a high concentration of low-income people of color. Lowrie, Solitare, and Himmelfarb (2011) also view brownfields from a community-assets perspective and the potential to bring communities together in their development.

Hoff, Mahfood, and McGuiness (2010, p. 20) go so far as to identify the tremendous potential of brownfields for urban agriculture:

Urban agriculture is a sustainable solution for brownfield sites that are not well positioned for immediate redevelopment. It embodies the three pillar definition of sustainability by enhancing environmental health, enabling economic profitability and by providing a food source to otherwise food insecure people in urban areas, it ensures social welfare and issues of equity that frequently surround redevelopment projects. It is not surprising, therefore that legislation and policy making at the federal level are favoring urban agriculture as a possible economically viable remedy at brownfield sites.

In addition to urban farming, these newly discovered places can incorporate physical changes to encourage physical exercise. They can be turned from blights to assets that benefit the entire community, including those who may use the spaces not for exercise but for socialization or beautification.

Schoolyards that are in disrepair and that are inaccessible to the public can be reclaimed for community physical activities (Hutch et al., 2011). The Boston Schoolyard Initiative, which represented a public-private partnership emphasizing community participation, converted schoolyards into community, educational, and political assets (Lopez, Campbell, and Jennings, 2008).

Receptivity of Places and Spaces

Proximity to urban parks and recreational facilities has been found to be influential for a healthy body mass index (BMI) (Wolch et al., 2011). Access to recreational facilities such as parks, however, depends upon a variety of factors that go beyond geography (Miyake, Maroko, Grady, Maantay, and Arno, 2010). Dahmann, Walch, Joassart-Marcelli, Reynolds, and Jerrett (2009), in a study of the spatial distribution of public recreational programs in Southern California, found significant disparities based on income, racial/ethnic composition, fiscal capacity, and multifamily dwellings, in access to these programs and in health risks, including obesity.

Having places and spaces for physical activity, such as playgrounds and parks, does not necessarily translate into community residents using such spaces. Loukaiton-Sideris (2006) highlights safety and security concerns and their influence on decisions about walking in the space. One North Carolina study found that restrictive school policies and fear of crime and danger were the primary barriers preventing youth from access to physical activity on a daily basis (Moore et al., 2010). An unsafe environment severely curtails any outdoor physical activity that is not essential.

Safety concerns, however, can go far beyond fear of crime, to encompass motor vehicle traffic and real or perceived dangers related to car accidents (Jacobson, Racioppi, and Rutter, 2009). Streets that are not safe for crossing (because they lack stop signs, working traffic lights, or policing to enforce driving laws) can become sites of pedestrian injuries and deaths, discouraging any form of walking that is not necessary (Perdue,

Stone, and Gostin, 2003). Marshall, Brauer, and Frank (2009) found that neighborhoods that are conducive for walking and have low exposure to pollution are rare in cities, and when present, they tend to be in high-income areas.

Mehta (2007, p. 167) advances a different perspective on city streets as social spaces, as opposed to venues for movement from one destination to another: "The findings reveal that people are equally concerned with the social, land use, and physical aspects of the street. Seating provided by businesses, seating provided by the public authorities, businesses that are community places, personalized street fronts, and sidewalk width particularly contribute to stationary and social activities on neighborhood commercial streets."

Urban places and spaces can exist to supplement the conventional views of parks and playgrounds as settings for physical exercise. Physical exercise interventions can also integrate nutritional changes in diets, opening up this arena for innovative advances that take into consideration context, both physical and cultural.

The CDC (Khan et al., 2009) recommends nine strategies for encouraging physical exercise. Communities should: (1) create safe environments that support physical activity; (2) improve access to outdoor recreational facilities; (3) enhance infrastructure supporting bicycling; (4) enhance infrastructure supporting walking; (5) support locating schools within easy walking distance of residential areas; (6) improve access to public transportation; (7) zone for mixed-use development; (8) enhance personal safety in areas where people are or could be physically active; and (9) enhance traffic safety in areas where people are or could be physically active.

Interventions to increase physical activity must be comprehensive and multifaceted, with short-, intermediate-, and long-term goals (Giles-Corti, 2006; Macintyre, Ellaway, and Cummins, 2002). Meyer (2008, p. 2) sums up this perspective: "In general, no single approach will solve the problem of obesity and physical activity. If a long-term, positive influence is to be exerted on the complex interaction between eating and exercise habits, a combination of behavioral/cognitive and political/environmental approaches is necessary."

We have seen how social forces can minimize physical exercise in marginalized urban communities. Low-income residents do not have access to safe areas to exercise. The streets are not conducive for walking. Parks and playgrounds, when available, are often considered unusable. Unlike their middle- and upper-middle-income counterparts, most low-income people of color cannot join health clubs.

It would be unfair to blame this nation's increase in overweight and obesity solely on higher calorie intake. Lack of physical exercise is a significant factor in the current trend toward excessive weight among so many Americans. However, a social justice perspective shifts a portion of the responsibility away from the individual and contributes to a more balanced understanding of the forces that minimize opportunities for engaging in physical exercise in a safe and supportive environment.

7

Food Industry Practices

Driven by this basic profit-above-all-else directive, corporations are mandated, in effect, to "grow or die," a rule also called "the growth imperative." Of course, a food maker is no different from any other corporation operating in a free economy. However, food companies face special challenges when it comes to obeying the market's growth imperative: because there's a limit—in theory, anyway—to the number of calories humans can consume, competition is especially fierce among food makers for the finite pool of money that consumers can spend.

(SIMON, 2006A, P. 5)

An in-depth examination of the social, economic, and political forces that operate in the food industry's advertising and marketing policies reveals how they foster overweight and obesity in the United States, working against a social justice agenda. The power of advertising and marketing in creating consumer demand for products cannot be overestimated, and low-income people of color in urban communities have been particularly targeted in this regard. Marketing and advertising are sometimes confused with each other. *Marketing* refers to activities that are coordinated to bring buyers and sellers together; *advertising* is one component of marketing, and takes the form of paid announcements (such as ads on television, in print media, and online) used to promote a product or service.

Freudenberg and Galea (2010) discuss how the world is becoming ever more urbanized, resulting in further concentrations of populations, and describe the increasing power (economic and political) of various corporations that sell products that undermine the health of urban-based population groups.

Food Industry Tactics

One of the greatest challenges is figuring out how the food industry seeks to subvert efforts at controlling unhealthy food practices. Understanding how the industry functions can help guide counter-efforts. Brownell and Horgen (2006) identified 12 common food industry tactics, summarized as follows:

1. Claiming sincere commitment to public health concerns: Issuing periodic announcements attesting to the importance of nutritional education and physical exercise programs.
2. Influencing public policy debates: Testifying at government hearings about the industry's commitment to improving the nation's physical fitness and nutrition.
3. Making campaign contributions to elected officials: Providing financial support to elected officials, particularly those on influential agricultural and nutrition committees, who hold favorable views of the industry and embrace a personal responsibility perspective.
4. Claiming that advertising is about market share and not consumption: Stressing the importance of maintaining market share, not increasing consumption of an unhealthy food product. Viewing the marketplace as a competitive arena and emphasizing that no company should be expected to compete with one hand tied behind its back.
5. Focusing attention on the importance of physical exercise: Emphasizing that lack of exercise is the primary reason for obesity. This tactic shifts the focus back to personal responsibility.
6. Steering attention away from food: This strategy includes a variety of obvious and not-so-obvious tactics, such as fighting efforts to introduce nutrition labels and complaining about how the food industry is singled out for punishment when people themselves are to blame for their obesity.
7. Claiming that there is no such thing as "good" or "bad" food: Emphasizing that it takes a total diet and not individual food items to cause weight gain and thus diverting attention away from select sectors of the industry, and specific items like sugary beverages.
8. Advocating against restrictive access: Some food industry representatives will argue that limiting access to certain foods (through taxation or banning them from schools, for example) undermines democracy and freedom of choice.

9. Advocating consumer choice: Similar to the preceding tactic; equating choices in food consumption with fundamental liberty.

10. Claiming that food regulations represent a "slippery slope": Raising concerns that limiting food choice may eventually lead to the undermining of other personal liberties.

11. Stating that it is a parental responsibility to teach children healthy eating habits: This perspective is very much along the lines of the personal responsibility argument.

12. Utilizing lawsuits and intimidation: Finally, the potential silencing of critics through legal actions claiming false statements, etc., is a way of exerting tremendous power to silence free speech.

The tactics summarized above illustrate the powerful arsenal that the food industry uses to address critics. When combined, they are quite formidable, particularly when they target marginalized communities that do not have representative government to advocate for their self-interests.

Marketing to Marginalized Communities

We live in an age dominated by media. Media can play a significant role in the creation of the crisis of overweight and obesity, as well as the crafting of solutions (Marshall, 2004; Samuels, Craypo, Lawrence, Lingas, and Dorfman, 2007).

In 1989, the Center for Science in the Public Interest (Maxwell and Jacobson, 1989) published a landmark study titled *Marketing Disease to Hispanics* as a follow-up to its book *Marketing Booze to Blacks* (Hacker, Collins, and Jacobson, 1987). These two studies highlighted, in very graphic ways, the challenges that Hispanic and black communities face in attempting to lead healthy lives. Since the publication of the two books, both population groups have increased in numbers, and so has their importance as a market for products and services, which explains why certain industries continue to target them (Delgado, 2011). Latinos, for example, account for half of the population growth in the United States since 2000, and this trend is expected to continue for the next several decades.

The tobacco industry is one industry that has embraced a variety of methods for marketing its products to marginalized communities. For example, tobacco corporate sponsorship is a highly visible marketing tool used by the industry. A 1995–1999 study (King and Siegel, 2001; Siegel, 2002) found that the tobacco industry sponsored 2,733 events during this period, at a cost of $365.4 million. Overall, sponsorship in North America increased from $850 million in 1985 to $7.6 billion in 1999. The marketing of menthol Kool cigarettes to the urban African American/black community is a powerful example of a campaign targeting urban-based population groups (Cruz, Wright, and Crawford, 2010). Marketing techniques that offer "two for the price of one" or "buy one and get the other free" are also not unusual in campaigns targeting low-income communities (Meyer, 2008).

Such tactics eventually brought the tobacco industry under fire. In 2009 President Obama signed the Family Smoking Prevention and Tobacco Control Act, which authorizes the FDA to regulate the manufacturing, marketing, distribution, sale, and importation of tobacco products (Dayton, Sharfstein, and Hamburg 2010). Unfortunately, advertising and marketing practices regarding unhealthy foods have not received the same level of regulation.

The deleterious consequences on the health of marginalized communities cannot be ignored if the public health of these groups is to be improved (Grier and Kumanyika, 2010, p. 349): "The use of marketing to connect products and services with consumers has increased and expanded over recent years. However, the pervasiveness and potential influence of advertising and other forms of marketing on consumer behavior and on sociocultural processes more generally continue to generate concerns, particularly as techniques change in ways that appear to extend marketing's influence, specificity, and reach."

Grier and Kumanyika (2008) found that African Americans are more vigorously targeted by marketing for high-caloric foods and drinks than are other groups. Billboards are placed in high-visibility areas in certain communities because of their strategic importance in reaching certain population groups. The clustering of unhealthy outdoor advertisements around child-serving institutions, for example, has been found to be positively associated with race (Hillier et al., 2009). More outdoor advertisements for unhealthy foods, like ads for alcohol and tobacco, are disproportionately found in poor, working-class communities of color than in middle- and upper-middle-class communities (Yancey et al., 2009).

Marketing to Children

The food industry uses a variety of methods to market unhealthy foods to children, in particular exploiting the power and influence of social media. In 2006 the food industry spent $11 billion advertising to children and adolescents, exposing them to approximately 40,000 food advertisements (Gostin, 2007). The importance of targeting this age group is significantly increased in Latino and African American communities because of the high concentration of youths (Elliott, 2011). The median age for white, non-Latinos is 41, but for Latinos, it is 27. In 2010, youth of color represented 48.5 percent of all those under the age of 18 (Tavernise, 2011b). Youth of color are projected to become the majority of youth by 2023. Furthermore, youth spend approximately 5.5 hours per day watching television or in front of a computer, making them easy targets for advertisements delivered through these media.

Roberts (2008, p. 104) makes an important distinction between food advertisements targeting children and those targeting adults: "Granted, adults see a lot of food ads, yet adults presumably have the cognitive capacity to judge accuracy and intent of ads; young children do not. Development experts say that before the age of eight, children lack the ability to understand the persuasive intent of ads and instead take their claims as truthful." Children wield considerable influence on family buying habits and are considered responsible for more than $100 billion a year in food and beverage expenditures, including more than half of all cold cereals bought in this country (Richtel, 2011).

In a rare study focused on Latino children, Arredondo, Castaneda, Elder, Slymen, and Dozier (2009) found that older children and children who are overweight had an increased level of recognition of fast-food restaurant logos as opposed to other food logos. On the basis of findings like this, Schmitt, Wagner, and Kirch (2007) recommend the passage of legislation that limits advertising aimed at children. However, Nordahl (2009, p. 41) suggests it is unlikely that such legislation will pass, and recommends other tactics: "Until then, healthy foods need to be just as visible and accessible as junk foods, preferably more so. Infusing our public spaces with fresh produce can help mitigate the marketing inundation of processed and fast foods, and actually teach children about the cycles of life, whole foods, and where those foods come from."

The food industry is quite creative in using advances in technology and social networking to directly target children without the intervention of their parents. Using social media such as Facebook pages, inserting quizzes on product packaging, and advertising on television, for example, are commonplace. A 2011 *New York Times* article about the use of online games as a marketing technique ("In Online Games, a Path to Young Consumers") shows how creative these strategies can be. Internet sites have also been developed by the fast-food industry as another way of targeting children and youth. Many companies use such sites to reach those age groups, among them General Mills (Lucky Charms, Trix, and Honey Nut Cheerios), Kellogg (Froot Loops and Apple Jacks), and Post (Fruity Pebbles and Cocoa Pebbles). These sites are certainly popular. McDonald's sites, including HappyMeal.com and McWorld.com, received 700,000 hits, with almost 50 percent from those under the age of 12, and General Mills's Lucky Charms site had 227,000 hits (Richtel, 2011). Critics and children's advocates have viewed such practices with alarm.

Richtel's (2011, p. A1) description of industry practices captures this challenge: "Like many marketers, General Mills and other food companies are rewriting the rules for reaching children in the Internet age. These companies, often selling sugar cereals and junk food, are using multimedia games, online quizzes and cellphone apps to build deep ties with young consumers. And children . . . are sharing their messages through e-mail and social networks, effectively acting as marketers."

The CDC recommends that communities exercise their powers to limit advertisements of less healthy foods and beverages (Khan et al., 2009).

In late April 2011, the FDC issued guidelines that covered a wide variety of current marketing efforts including television, print ads, Internet sites, online games, product placements in movies, and the use of movie characters in cross-productions and fast-food children's meals (Neuman, 2011). The FDC guidelines, however, are meant to be voluntary, with a goal of having participating companies reach compliance within a five-to–ten-year period. These guidelines have two primary goals: (1) increase the consumption of healthy ingredients and (2) eliminate the use of unhealthy amounts of sodium, sugar, trans fat, and saturated fat (Neuman, 2011).

Parents do have the ultimate responsibility for their children's eating behaviors. One study of Latino parents with children in Head Start showed high levels of ability to prevent obesity through their influences on meals (Glassman, Figueroa, and Irigoyen, 2011). However, pitching advertising messages directly to children can create tension in the home when parents and their children differ about what is in the children's best health interest. Goren, Harris, Schwartz, and Brownell (2010), not surprisingly, found support from parents, particularly parents who had concerns about current food practices, about restricting unhealthy food marketing to youths. These findings support public education campaigns that highlight how food industry marketing influences eating habits among youth and the important role that parents can play in limiting the influence of these messages.

Can we fight Madison Avenue? The answer is yes, we can. It is clear that any fight against overweight and obesity in marginalized communities is not a fair fight when the food industry, its lobbyists, and the elected officials depending upon it for contributions have no vested interest in looking out for the marginalized, whose political support is not counted upon. A personal responsibility approach is a smoke screen; a social justice perspective provides the social work profession with sufficient justification to make its influence heard at the national and state levels, and in coalitions and task forces opposing this industry's policies and practices.

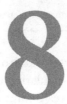

Challenges in
Measuring Overweight and Obesity

Standardizing our weights. Now some may question why this is a very
big deal; after all, does it really matter if the government gets its weight
standards exactly right? . . . First, being classified as overweight has an
immediate impact on the lives of millions of Americans: it can determine whether they can work at certain jobs, whether they are considered fit parents, or whether certain drugs or medical procedures will
be paid by insurance or tax money.

(OLIVER, 2006, PP. 33–34)

The average person could not imagine how arduous it is to accurately
measure overweight and obesity; in fact, the terms are often used interchangeably, even though they technically refer to two very different
conditions. We will now turn to identifying the challenges and rewards
associated with how we measure the problem of excessive weight, and
the difficulties in arriving at a consensus. Failure to reach a consensus,
however, will lead to fragmented and ultimately unsuccessful programs
to combat the issue.

If we are calibrating our prescription devices based on incorrect measurements, we have little hope of solving the obesity epidemic. As individuals, we will fail to alter the behaviors that make us fat. By putting
our energy and money into the wrong diets and lifestyle changes, we will
neglect that the environment is itself the product of manipulation. State
and national policies will similarly fail to eliminate our collective spare
tire because they, too, will be aimed disproportionately at the individual.

(BENFORADO, HANSON, AND YOSIFON, 2006, P. 1653)

Similarly, Evans and Colls (2009) point out the detrimental consequences
of relying on body mass index (BMI) as the standard measurement tool
in anti-obesity initiatives.

Gray (unpublished manuscript), lists three key definitional challenges: (1) the rise of a global definition of obesity ("globesity"); (2) the use of body mass index (BMI) as a measurement tool, despite its measurement discrepancies across several populations; and (3) methodological complications in collecting data.

Burkhauser and Cawley (2008, p. 519), sum up the need for more accurate measures of excess weight in research:

> In the long run, social science datasets should include more accurate measures of fatness. In the short run, estimating more accurate measures of fatness using height and weight is not possible except by making unattractive assumptions, but there is also no reason to adhere uncritically to BMI as a measure of fatness. Social science research on obesity would be enriched by greater consideration of alternate specifications of weight and height and more accurate measures of fatness.

Numerous conceptual and methodological challenges impede our understanding of overweight and obesity as a social, behavioral, psychological, genetic, and biologic phenomenon, making research into the topic extremely complex (Booth, Pinkston, and Poston, 2005; Hu, 2008). These challenges, incidentally, were recognized and reported almost 15 years ago (Allison et al., 1998), yet minimal progress has been achieved since then. In 2001 Jebb and Prentice suggested the need for a consensus definition of what constitutes an overweight or obese individual. That definition, unfortunately, is still elusive, although a cadre of critics is forcing serious deliberations and making progress.

Not surprisingly, a lack of agreement on a definition makes national and international comparisons difficult. It also encourages a propensity to inflate the numbers of overweight and obese individuals within a given population.

BMI as a Weight Measurement Tool

The body mass index (BMI) measure was created by Adolphe Quetelet, a Belgian statistician, in 1832; it was not originally developed to study obesity but rather to study human physical characteristics (Cut the Waist, 2009). In 1997 the World Health Organization (WHO), after preliminary work of the International Obesity Task Force, officially declared the need for a global definition and standardized measure, and adopted the body mass index (James, Jackson-Leach, and Rigby, 2010). A weight classification system was recommended for international use, with the labeling of 25 kilograms (55 pounds) as class I (at risk for developing health-related problems) as overweight, 30 kilograms (66 pounds) as class II (at high risk for developing health-related problems) as obese, and 40 kilograms (88 pounds) as class III (morbidly obese, at extreme risk for developing health-related problems and even death). These cutoff points have been labeled as arbitrary by some scholars (James, 2008; Mascie-Taylor and Goto, 2007; Stommel and Schoenborn, 2010). Yet their importance, for employment and insurance purposes, for example, is immense. Nevertheless, a year after the WHO report was released, the National Institutes of Health (NIH) provided clinical guidelines for the identification, evaluation, and treatment of overweight and obesity.

BMI is widely considered a "surrogate" for measuring body fat percentage. What is the most effective way of measuring body fat? Kuczmarski (2007) argues that the only effective way to truly measure body fat is through the use of chemical analysis of cadavers, which obviously would be highly impractical from a prevention and treatment perspective. Thus, only indirect methods of measurement are viable. The importance of a standardized measure cannot be overestimated from a public health perspective, and particularly a measure that is practical, non-intrusive, quick, relatively inexpensive, and easy to use (Fogli, 2005; Thompson, 2008).

BMI is generally correlated with body fat but does not actually measure fat itself or, for that matter, where the fat is stored. Further, it does not account for skeletal size, muscle mass, water retention, or gender (European Union Public Health System, 2009). Two individuals with the same BMI can have very different distribution of body fat, with dramatically different health statuses. BMI can overestimate body fat content in individuals who are very muscular and underestimate it in individuals who have lost muscle mass, such as older adults. Body builders, for example, may have BMI ratings that would classify them as "overweight," but their scores are the result of high muscle mass and heavier bone structure. Long-distance runners, on the other hand, may have BMI measures that would classify them as underweight, and therefore unhealthy. Being of "typical" weight, however, does not automatically translate into a healthy state either! The use of BMI in children and pregnant women, too, has serious limitations.

Another primary criticism of BMI from a global perspective is the overreliance on research findings from an almost exclusive use in Western populations (Ogden, Yanovski, Carroll, and Flegal, 2007; World Health Organization, 2000). The conclusions based on these findings, in turn, get applied to non-Western nations. Asian countries have raised serious concerns about the use of BMI standards that have little applicability to their population groups, and have argued for lower cutoff points on the basis of their own research (Rush, Freitas, and Plank, 2009; WHO Expert Consultation, 2004).

In response to this criticism, a 2004 World Health Organization report called for countries to develop their own public health action plans specifically tailored to their populations. These action plans also needed to acknowledge differences involving ethnicity, BMI, and health consequences. No uniform system exists as this book goes to press (WHO Expert Consultation, 2004). Consequently, it is still difficult, if not impossible, to make international comparisons.

Mascie-Taylor and Goto (2007, p. 109) provide a reasoned, yet scathing critique of the use of BMI:

> The method used to establish BMI cut-offs has been largely arbitrary and has been based on the visual inspection of the relationship between BMI and mortality whereby the cut-off of 30 relates to a point of flexion of the curve. However a number of studies on BMI and mortality have methodological drawbacks (such as failure to control for cigarette smoking and to eliminate early mortality) and most have been conducted on people living in Western Europe or the USA.

A number of scholars have also argued that the use of BMI and the categorization resulting from these measures, such as "normal," "overweight," and "obese," for example, can be considered capricious in relation to the five most prevalent health risks associated with obesity: hypertension, type 2 diabetes, chronic heart disease, asthma, and arthritis (Stommel and Schoenborn, 2009).

This classification, in addition, has a specific detrimental impact on marginalized population groups, further stigmatizing those who are "overweight" or "obese," raising the role of social justice in understanding and addressing this phenomenon of stigmatization. There is a need to take into account variations by race/ethnicity, age, gender, and socioeconomic status regarding BMI, and corresponding body fat to avoid misclassification of overweight and obesity (Burkhauser and Cawley, 2008; Mascie-Taylor and Goto, 2007; Ogden et al., 2007).

Given all the limitations raised by the use of BMI, the search for alternative methods has started to gain traction. Chaoyand, Ford, McGuire, and Mokdad (2007) argue that abdominal obesity may be a more effective predictor than overall obesity for disease risks and mortality. Precise measurement of abdominal fat necessitates the use of radiological imaging technology, which is expensive. Consequently, waist circumference (w.c.) is recommended as an alternative method for measuring abdominal fat mass. Unfortunately, as Ross and colleagues (2008) note, there is not even a consensus on the optimal protocol for measuring waist circumference.

Peltz, Aguirre, Sanderson, and Fadden (2010), in a study of Mexican men and women, compared BMI, PBF (percent body fat), and FMI (fat mass index), and found FMI to be a more accurate measure for determining obesity. Bergman and colleagues (2011), in turn, recommend the use of a body adiposity index (BAI), which relies upon height and hip circumference measurements. Others have found the measurement of skin folds, or surface anthropometry to be an effective method (Nevill, Stewart, Olds, and Holder, 2006).

Himes (2009, p. 3), in reviewing a variety of weight measures for use with children, concluded that BMI is the preferred method: "There is little evidence that other measures of body fat such as skinfolds, waist circumference, or bioelectrical impedance are sufficiently practicable or provide appreciable added information to be used in the identification of children and adolescents who are overweight or obese." Nafiu and colleagues (2010), however, recommend using neck circumference in children as a simple and effective technique, with good inter-rater reliability (the degree to which independent coders arrive at the same conclusion).

Obesity Measurement in Various Populations

Lissner (2002) examines a wide range of problems with measuring obesity along various dimensions (race and ethnicity, age, gender, and socioeconomic status). His concerns have implications for any form of health promotion or prevention intervention that stresses food intake.

Race and Ethnicity

The importance of race and ethnicity cannot be overlooked in any effort to better understand overweight and obesity (Kumanyika, 2008b). Kuczmarski (2007, p. 32) sums up issues regarding BMI measurement among people of color: "There are important differences that influence both the relative utility of abdominal circumference or BMI as indicators of health risk as well as the definition of obesity using these measures."

Burkhauser and Cawley (2008) state that use of BMI as an obesity measure significantly misclassifies African Americans as obese when compared to the more accurate measure of percentage of body fat, which is the result of genetic differences in muscle, bone, and fluid. Not surprisingly, the role of racism in this form of classification emerges. The stigmatization that results from being labeled as obese further marginalizes African Americans and other groups of color, severely affecting their employment options and possibility of obtaining high-quality health care.

Kumanyika (2008b, p. 586) sums up the need for more research on interventions, obesity, and people of color:

> Yet, the evidence-based experience with obesity interventions is still rudimentary as it relates to ethnic minorities in the population at large. We should continue to ask the question of "what works in minority populations," but we should ask it with greater clarity as to the types of information needed to derive useful answers. Efforts to improve the relevance and quality of evidence on obesity prevention and treatment to a more diverse set of populations will improve the relevance and quality of the weight control literature as a whole.

Kumanyika's charge to the field will necessitate a more nuanced understanding and approach to community-based interventions.

Age

The need for definitions that are specific to select age groups is particularly important in addressing all stages of the life cycle and in the development of age-appropriate interventions, especially for children, youth, and adolescents. These age categories are far too broad for the purposes of effectively targeted interventions. Adolescence, for example, covers a six-year period (from age 13 to 19). The developmental needs and understanding of what excessive weight signifies will vary considerably over those years.

The importance of accurately measuring overweight and obesity among young populations cannot be overstated. Irigoyen, Glassman, Chen, and Findley (2008) found that early-childhood overweight and obesity have reached alarming levels among low-income urban children of color in New York City (more than 50 percent are either overweight or obese by their fifth birthday). Kimbro, Brooks-Gunn, and McLanahan (2006), in a national sample of 3-year-olds in urban and low-income families, found that 35 percent of the children were either overweight or obese. More specifically, Latino children were twice as likely as either black or white, non-Latino children to be among that 35 percent. Latino children with mothers who were obese were at particular risk.

Jebb and Prentice (2001, p. 999) raise concerns about the standards that have been established to determine overweight and obesity among children:

> Firstly, different values are obtained according to which centile standards are used, which makes international comparisons impossible. Secondly, the true nature of secular trends are obscured if updated standards are used; these standards are themselves affected by the developing epidemic of obesity (leading ultimately to the self fulfilling prophecy that there will always be 15% overweight and 5% obesity if these cut-off points are applied to contemporary standards). Thirdly, the choice of 85th and 95th centiles effectively inflates the apparent number of overweight and obese children. This has led to confusion over the prevalence of obesity in young people.

Older adults also face challenges regarding overweight and obesity. Unfortunately, there is a paucity of research involving older adults; current standards for BMI cutoffs are based largely on studies of young and middle-aged adults (Corrada and Paganini-Hill, 2010). This age bias limits our understanding of excessive weight among this age group, and is particularly acute among older adults of color (Delgado, 2008).

Advocates for the use of BMI argue that the field is evolving and it is only a question of time before extensive studies involving older adults and other groups will be undertaken. Critics, however, argue that standards based upon research findings of one age group should not be extended to other groups. An embrace of social justice principles must translate into measures that are sensitive to the factors that make certain groups particularly at risk for overweight and obesity.

Gender

The subject of weight and gender is a sensitive topic. In this society women who are overweight or obese are more stigmatized than are men with the same profile. Utilizing the same BMI classifications for men and women causes an even greater over-classification of body fat in women and an even greater under-classification of body fat in men (Ogden et al., 2007), thus biasing any discussion concerning overweight toward women, who in general are much more sensitive about their weight.

Socioeconomic Status (SES)

Low-income and low-wealth communities have increased access to fast-food establishments, limited access to healthy food, and limited options for physical exercise. The BMI measurement places its entire emphasis on individuals and fails to take into account such social forces (Connelly and Ross, 2007). Consequently, measures that are individualistic need to be complemented by measures that are ecological as a way of balancing the picture regarding overweight and obesity among poor and working-class groups, which invariably tend to be people of color. Shifting the emphasis to population groups also increases the feasibility of using a social justice perspective to develop a better understanding of the forces restraining their search for healthier lifestyles related to food consumption and exercise.

Methodological Challenges

All classification systems bring with them inherent advantages and disadvantages. The limitations of a classification system that relies on BMI are considerable. However, the field also faces a number of challenges related to methodology, three of which will be addressed in more detail here: (1) reliance on self-reported data, (2) cultural norms and variations, and (3) over-reliance on quantitative data.

1. Reliance on Self-Reporting: Self-reports of height and weight are unquestionably one of the most popular ways for getting data on BMI (Gorber, Treblay, Moher, and Gorber, 2006). This method has several

advantages: it is not invasive or expensive to administer, and it provides consumers with a voice in determining their BMI status, which is quite empowering.

However, Rothman (2008) critiques the use of BMI as a measure of obesity when it is based on self-reported height and weight. One Canadian study (Shields, Gorber, and Tremblay, 2008) found that both men and women tended to over-report their heights and under-report their weights, particularly when the respondents were overweight or obese. When weight and height were measured, the prevalence of obesity was 9 percent higher among males and 6 percent higher among women.

The age of the respondent has also been found to influence the results. Seghers and Claessens (2010) found that children ages 8–11 were not able to accurately estimate their height and weight.

The method used to ask a respondent about height and weight also has an impact on BMI results. Ezzati, Martin, Skjold, Hoom, and Murray (2006), for example, note that data obtained over the telephone can be significantly less valid than that gathered in person.

2. Cultural Norms and Values: Shared food preferences and eating behaviors are essential elements of a cultural construct (Bramble, Cornelius, and Simpson, 2009; Larson and Story, 2009). Ten Eyck (2007) advocates using a cultural lens to develop a deeper understanding of overweight and obesity, instead of the current emphasis on either social forces or individual choices. Weight is a social phenomenon and its sociocultural context, is influenced accordingly. However, the field of overweight and obesity has only recently started to entertain the possibility that cultural norms and values play a compounding role in how weight is viewed and, in the case of excessive weight, how best to address it.

Normative bias (a propensity to report what is culturally expected) is one of the key factors that need to be considered in any attempt to measure overweight and obesity (Lissner, 2002). The influence of cultural and ethnic/racial background of respondents plays a critical role in determining their perceptions of weight (Phelan, 2009). One study of urban parents' estimates of their children's weight found that many parents do underestimate their children's weight and are not concerned about excessive weight (Tschamier, Conn, Cook, and Halterman, 2009). Erroneous perceptions of weight and height, however, may reflect a sign of resiliency to buffer against society's stigmatizing labels of undervalued groups. In other words, "excessive" weight has symbolic meaning depending upon the cultural context.

There is a relationship between higher socioeconomic status and low body weight preference. This SES standard, however, represents a narrow, although powerful, sector of this society.

Bennett and Wolin (2006) found that African Americans were 50 percent more likely than white, non-Latinos to misrepresent their weight, and Latinos were 70 percent more likely. Davidson and Knafi (2006) found that white, non-Latinos viewed excessive weight as unattractive, while other racial and ethnic groups saw it as positive and attractive.

Bramble, Cornelius, and Simpson (2009) examine eating as a form of cultural expression among Afro-Caribbean and African American women, and stress the importance of not generalizing to entire groups on the basis of limited samples. Kumanyika (2008a) also notes that the role of culture and beliefs in influencing diet can be quite strong; it must be part of any knowledge base on the subject and be incorporated into initiatives. Christie, Watkins, Weerts, and Jackson (2010) examine the role of religion in the lives of African American women and the potential of church-based interventions. Robertson (2011) describes the potential role that African American preachers could play in promoting healthy diets in certain regions of the country.

3. Quantitative Bias: The field of overweight and obesity is dominated by quantitative research and reliance on a limited number of national data sets, which offer a very narrow perspective on a complicated social phenomenon. This situation ultimately results in findings from dominant social groups being used as social indicators of overweight and obesity for all groups. A social justice perspective would call for the development of measures that have been qualitatively grounded. Such measures would provide a more realistic picture of what excessive weight means to various groups rather than relying upon an inaccurate picture imposed by those most removed from the community.

Brown (1992) advocates the use of popular epidemiological efforts in which community members actively pursue scientific knowledge in an effort to control a social problem. This perspective both empowers the participants and serves to engage communities in shaping discourse and solutions to local problems. Corburn (2009) argues that community residents should have an active and prominent role in determining the health status classification of their communities. This can be done in partnership with researchers who value their insights.

Excessive reliance on a limited number of quantitative studies further exacerbates the development of a comprehensive picture of overweight and obesity of marginalized communities in this country. The National

Health and Nutrition Examination Survey (NHANES) can be labeled the "poster child" for data on national health trends in the United States, including overweight and obesity. However, this survey reports only on broad racial/ethnic categories, such as "non-Hispanic Whites," "non-Hispanic Blacks," and "Mexican Americans," which severely limits its usefulness from a social intervention perspective (Bates, Acevedo-Garcia, Alegria, and Krieger, 2008; CDC, 2010c).

The ever-popular CDC growth chart was developed relying only on the NHANES I and II from the 1960s, the NHANES I and II from the 1970s, and the NHANES III from the early 1990s (CDC, 2010a). This reliance—or as some critics would argue, over-reliance—on those particular measures favors a single-data-point approach to data collection, whereas the complexity of overweight and obesity necessitates a multifaceted approach that utilizes qualitative as well as quantitative measures.

Qualitative measures are very much needed in order to develop a conceptually more sound grounding for the meaning of weight, its distribution on the human body, and the most culturally competent ways of addressing excessive weight and the diseases caused by it. Further, these qualitative measures must also be sensitive to urban environmental factors and considerations. Overweight and obesity interventions must be contextually based, a goal that renders broad-based quantitative measures of limited use.

The Need for New Measurement Methods

It is fitting to issue a call here for new methods and standards for determining excessive weight. A social phenomenon such as excessive weight is complex, and thus necessitates a combination of different perspectives if we are to obtain a more comprehensive and in-depth understanding of its root causes and potential solutions (Dijkum, 2000; Suarez-Balcazar et al., 2006).

Flegal and Ogden (2011, p. 1595) address the importance of a consensus definition:

> Definitions of overweight and obesity are generally statistical rather than risk-based and use a variety of different reference data sets for BMI. As a result, different definitions often do not give the same results. A basic problem is the lack of strong evidence for any one particular definition. Rather than formulate the question as being one of how to define obesity,

it might be useful to consider what BMI cut-points best predict future health risks and how efficiently to screen for such risks. The answers may be different for different populations.

The authors, nevertheless, still see BMI as a practical measure.

The appeal of BMI is quite strong because it is easy to use, it has a long history, and it is widely accepted in the scientific community. There would be a tremendous amount of resistance to setting aside BMI as the "industry standard" for use in the field of obesity studies and practice. However, like universal measurements, which strive to set normative standards, it cannot be all things to all people, particularly when it is applied to racial and ethnic groups.

The reader may wonder what this charge has to do with social work. The medical profession is probably the biggest champion of the use of BMI. The social work profession, however, must not fall into the trap of developing interventions that are based upon the use of BMI, and must be critical of interventions predicated exclusively on this measure.

Any new methods of measurement and standards for excessive weight categories must incorporate the following four principles if they are to have any degree of relevance among marginalized subgroups such as low-income people of color residing in the nation's cities:

1. They must be relatively easy to implement (low-cost and non-intrusive). Some of the methods that have emerged as alternatives to the BMI hold much promise but are not easy to implement. Ease of implementation may be more valuable than precision of outcome. The issue of excessive weight among particular subgroups is not a question of one or two pounds' making a difference. Thus, the precise measurement of weight to the ounce or pound is not necessary.

2. The measure must take into account the meaningful input (experiential knowledge) of the marginalized subgroups that it intends to assess (Corburn, 2005, 2009). Weight is a socially constructed measure and subject to a host of biases that relate to social, economic, and cultural forces. A twenty-first-century effort at measurement must not rely on a nineteenth-century tool.

3. The meaning of any weight-related study results must be contextualized to the local community where the assessment was conducted. Standardized measures are attractive because they can be applied across all population groups regardless of setting. However, these practices, al-

though attractive for comparison and cost purposes, are counterproductive for contextualized interventions.

4. The meaning of excessive weight once measured, and determined, must be grounded within the context and groups it is based upon. In essence, there is no universal reaction to weight. Interventions must therefore take into account local circumstances and expectations. Broad categories or parameters may eventually be determined to draw a more comprehensive picture of weight than the limited categories that we currently use ("overweight," "obese," "excessive obesity").

These four principles will not be attractive to most scientists and scholars. However, it is apparent that the current method of using BMI and the weight categories that result do serious harm to marginalized groups in this country. There is tension between generalizing findings across groups and grounding findings within very specific or contextualized locales and all major groups and sub-groups. I hope that implementation of the above principles will help to minimize these tensions.

A consensus on how best to measure overweight and obesity is of immense importance, yet it has been, and continues to be, a challenge for the field. Without a widely agreed-upon measure, it is difficult to determine what constitutes excessive weight and what its consequences are. A consensus definition must also take into account social, economic, cultural, and political factors.

While BMI is considered the "gold standard" from which interventions are developed, other methods are slowly emerging in an effort to increase the validity of measurement options for excessive weight.

The scientific community clearly "owns" the definition of overweight and obesity and the tools used to measure it. Communities are rarely, if ever, consulted as to their own definitions and preferred methods for measuring excessive weight. Such a "top-down" approach is not only disempowering but also misses the opportunity to contextualize weight and to identify the most appropriate methods for achieving significant and healthy weight loss for those who wish to lose weight.

Some critics, including this author, see a reliance upon a measure that is weak when applied to marginalized groups from a social justice perspective. Any measure that systematically undermines a particular group, such as those who are of color and fall into the lower strata of society, cannot be considered just.

2

Community-Led Health Promotion Approaches

9

Health Promotion

Should a community defer to professionals, trusting that the findings
are accurate and that they are sharing all the information they have?
Do professionals have an obligation to take into account community-
generated information and to incorporate it, somehow, into their formal analyses? Should local accounts of health risk ever trump expert
knowledge? Can we imagine a situation in which we should not put
our lives and community well-being in the hands of technical experts?
(CORBURN, 2005, P. 3)

Corburn's quote sums up the social justice health promotion model that,
I believe, the social work profession must embrace in addressing overweight and obesity in undervalued or marginalized communities.

This chapter offers a more detailed definition of health promotion and
also identifies a set of values and principles, grounds health promotion
interventions in a socioecological perspective, and explores the challenges in using evidence- and evaluation-based practice research. Each of
these perspectives wields prodigious influence in how health promotion
is conceived, implemented, and eventually evaluated for the overweight
and obesity field.

As already noted, health can and should be grounded in a sociopolitical
context, utilizing multidisciplinary approaches and social justice values
(Baum, 2007; King, Vigil, Herrera, Hajek, and Jones, 2007). Social work
has much to contribute to this method because of its emphasis on socioecological theories, community, marginalized groups, urban practice,
empowerment, and capacity enhancement (Delgado, 2009; Delgado and
Zhou, 2008).

Morgan and Ziglio (2007) observe that population health promotion has traditionally been based on a deficit (medical) model, providing a narrow and disempowering perspective. The adoption of an assets

model instead opens up the field of health promotion to exciting public health developments. Communities and individuals who are overweight or obese have a significant role to play in this movement toward social justice, including community capacity enhancement (Kegler, Rigler, and Honeycutt, 2011).

The most promising health promotion interventions actively seek to tap local knowledge and community participation in all phases of the intervention (Lorenc, Harden, Brunton, and Oakley, 2008). Further, these efforts embrace the values of enhancing community capacity in the process of addressing local health concerns. This conceptualization lends itself quite readily to social work contributions for the evolution of health promotion. A holistic perspective on excessive weight gain that is grounded in a social justice viewpoint resonates for the profession.

Definition of Health Promotion

Health promotion can view health from a broad perspective, one that includes social justice. The definition that guides this book was developed in 1986 at the World Health Organization's First International Conference on Health Promotion, held in Ottawa, Canada:

> Health promotion is the process of enabling people to increase control over, and to improve, their health. To reach a state of complete physical, mental and social well-being, an individual or group must be able to identify and to realize aspirations, to satisfy needs, and to change or cope with the environment. Health is, therefore, seen as a resource for everyday life, not the objective of living. Health is a positive concept emphasizing social and personal resources, as well as physical capacities. Therefore, health promotion is not just the responsibility of the health sector, but goes beyond healthy life-styles to well-being.

The Ottawa conference (Perkins, 2009; Raphael, 2006) was followed by the 2005 World Health Organization conference that established the Commission on Social Determinants of Health, validating the grounding of health in a broad social context and further pushing the definition of health beyond the conventional physical sphere. These two conferences significantly shaped how health promotion is conceptualized, building upon a social justice foundation, and they will continue to shape the evolution of this form of social intervention. Social work, too, has embraced social determinants of health perspectives, facilitating engagement in multidisciplinary, community-focused efforts (Moniz, 2010) and bringing us into close contact and possible collaboration with the public health profession.

Values Guiding Health Promotion

Social values are the foundation of any social intervention or helping profession. Sometimes these values are explicit; at other times they are implicit. Regardless, these values influence how academics and practitioners view the subject of overweight and obesity. The social values addressed here will resonate with the social justice paradigm discussed earlier. Here I will also stress the need to incorporate the values of those who are overweight and obese, as they are the ultimate beneficiaries of health promotion interventions.

Indigenous or cultural values are often either overlooked or minimized in health interventions. Capturing a sense of cultural values can be an arduous task. Nevertheless, cultural values play an influential role in determining whether overweight or obesity is considered a "health problem" and if it is, how best to address it in a non-stigmatizing manner.

For example, the Latino Coalition for a Healthy California (2006, p. 5) advocates that cultural context be considered in informing health promotion interventions: "Therefore, health promotion efforts in Latino communities will likely benefit from a focus on family involvement, strengthening of social networks, and development of social support. . . . The creation of social networks is particularly important among immigrants who may otherwise be marginalized and disengaged from civic action." This statement can also apply to other racial and ethnic groups.

Health promotion initiatives targeting overweight and obesity must adopt models that take into account the unique circumstances and demographic profiles of those they wish to reach (Budrys, 2003; Fitzpatrick and LaGory, 2000). Health promotion should also take into account the social and economic forces shaping health and illness with communities, and the responses (or lack thereof) of the organizations set up to address these illnesses.

Not surprisingly, the field of health promotion has enjoyed a dramatic increase in attention, both nationally and internationally, because of its promise for addressing health-related issues in all population groups.

Principles Guiding Health Promotion

I have always been a big fan of using principles in the development of community interventions. Principles fulfill a variety of important functions. First and foremost, they serve as a vital bridge between theory and practice, aiding practitioners in translating theoretical concepts into action. Probably one of the greatest criticisms leveled at academics is their inability to facilitate translation of theory and research findings into practice. Principles, I believe, help us achieve this transition. The field of obesity prevention has started to develop best-practice principles for addressing community-based interventions (King, Gill, Allender, and Swinburn, 2011).

Principles, in addition, draw upon values that we rely on to guide us. As social workers we are certainly not new to understanding how values shape interventions, weight-related or otherwise. Consequently, health promotion principles represent an amalgamation of values and theory. In reality, we cannot separate the two, even though we often write about theory as if it were value-free. Health promotion can never be considered value-free. It is important, therefore, to articulate our biases as clearly as possible. Health promotion principles, I believe, do this in an effective way.

Delgado and Zhou (2008) identified 11 health promotion principles, which since have been updated and collapsed into eight that specifically address the subject of overweight and obesity. These principles are not intended as a "menu" from which practitioners can pick and choose; they should be viewed as a "package deal," so to speak, in order to maximize the impact of weight-focused interventions.

King, Gill, Allender, and Swinburn (2011, p. 328), however, issue a caveat that applies to the principles that follow:

It is important to recognize that the full set of best practice principles is aspirational, and that it is not possible to specify a hierarchy of principles or a threshold level of adoption. In practice, the application of each component principle is context-specific and will vary according to such factors as the nature and size of the community, as well as organizational factors, including the resources and capacity available to support implementation.

In essence, principles are far from being a cookbook recipe, which invariably is very detailed and thus prescriptive in character.

The eight principles that follow are generally descriptive rather than prescriptive in character.

1. Community assets must form the foundation upon which we develop interventions focused on excessive weight. No community, regardless of how marginalized or undervalued, is without assets. Health promotion must actively seek to identify indigenous resources and build interventions that enhance them in the process of addressing overweight and obesity. Assets must be the initial component of any equation, followed by needs. Both are essential to understanding the meaning and extent of overweight and obesity in a community.

The process of identifying and engaging community assets is as important as the end result of a successful intervention. These assets, however, are not standardized, and careful assessment is required to determine their significance and potential role in a health promotion project, taking into account a sociocultural understanding and local circumstances.

2. Community participation must be stressed throughout all facets of an intervention. Ultimate ownership of a health promotion project must rest in the hands of the community it seeks to address. Consequently, communities represent an essential element in the planning, implementation, and evaluation of these efforts, and avenues for community participation must be included in all phases of an overweight or obesity intervention.

Participatory democratic principles represent a core dimension of health promotion projects that seek to empower communities. Weight-related projects, too, must stress participation at all levels of an intervention. Participation can be conceptualized along a continuum, with each stage representing greater and greater involvement and ownership. However, local circumstances and the community's history of involvement must be taken into account when planning participation if maximum benefits and experiences are to be ensured.

3. Inclusiveness must be a cornerstone of overweight and obesity interventions. Communities consist of many different groups, and even urban communities of color are not monolithic. Health promotion must seek to

include all significant sectors. Very few groups in marginalized communities are able to escape excessive weight and its consequences. Therefore, the more that weight-related intervention strategies take an inclusive approach, the more meaningful they become.

Bringing together key subgroups in a community also serves to increase the likelihood that interventions avoid the error of viewing a geographical area as monolithic without considering the needs of various subgroups.

4. Interventions must be sufficiently flexible to accommodate local circumstances. It would be unreasonable to expect health promotion strategies to be standardized to the point that they could be transported to and applied anywhere in the country. These strategies must be sufficiently flexible to take into account local conditions and circumstances to increase their effectiveness. Strategies that may be effective with a population that consists of American citizens, for example, will need to be modified to reach out to communities that are primarily undocumented.

5. Overweight and obesity must be addressed at multiple levels. The complexity of overweight and obesity can best be appreciated and addressed only through the use of a socioecological model. This model requires that social workers and other helping professions address root causes through a focus at the community level without ever losing sight of the individuals and their families.

An ecological model brings to the fore the need to be comprehensive in order to avoid failure and the blaming of the victim. We must make sure that we do not stigmatize communities because of the prevalence of excessive weight. Addressing the problem of excessive weight at multiple levels helps to ensure that individuals are not blamed for lack of access to healthy foods or to physical space that is conducive to exercise.

6. Interventions must avoid the "personal responsibility" trap. Health promotion initiatives must eschew being predicated on the personal responsibility argument advocated by the food industry. The forces that affect urban low-income communities of color go far beyond individual choice. Developing interventions that stress personal responsibility will reinforce a "blaming the victim" scenario.

The lack of physical or financial access to healthy foods, the overabundance of unhealthy foods, and the lack of access to safe spaces in which to exercise make it unfair to blame residents of these communities for not exercising enough or for not eating wholesome and healthy foods.

7. Health promotion interventions must identify indigenous leaders and support them in leadership roles. Every community, regardless of

how marginalized it is, possesses individuals who adopt leadership roles and also individuals who have the potential to do so now and in the future. Youth, for example, fall into this category. Thus interventions must seek to identify current and potential future leaders.

8. Health promotion interventions must seek to enter into all segments of a community and not just focus on the formal aspects of community life. Residents eat, play, work, worship, and socialize in communities. Overweight and obesity interventions must permeate all facets of community life. This principle will require the development of innovative approaches toward helping residents embrace a healthier lifestyle. Public education campaigns, for example, must tap the primary sources from which residents receive their information. Mainstream media may not be the preferred route in getting information on excessive weight into a community; for example, any campaign aiming to reach youth would likely want to explore the use of social media.

Health Promotion Framework

Frameworks help practitioners operationalize theory and principles in a manner that lends itself to actual use. There are numerous frameworks that social workers and other helping professionals can draw upon to develop community-focused overweight and obesity interventions. Swinburn, Gill, and Kumanyika (2005, p. 23), for example, propose a framework that facilitates translating evidence into action: "The framework is defined by five key policy and programme issues that form the basis of the framework. These are: (i) building a case for action on obesity; (ii) identifying contributing factors and points of intervention; (iii) defining the opportunities for action; (iv) evaluating potential interventions; and (v) selecting a portfolio of specific policies, programmes, and actions."

Stokols, Green, Leischow, Holmes, and Buchholz (2003), in turn, advance a framework that emphasizes development of community partnerships and brings together four models: (1) social ecology (which emphasizes the role of the environment in shaping expectations and behaviors); (2) life course health development, or LCHD (which focuses on biological and behavioral mechanisms throughout the life span that influence health trajectories); (3) Predisposing, Reinforcing, and Enabling Constructs in Educational Diagnosis and Evaluation (PRECEDE) and Policy, Regulatory, and Organizational Constructs in Educational and Environmental

Development (PROCEED) (a participatory process that seeks to close the gap between health promotion research and practice by drawing upon systems theory); and (4) community partnering (which emphasizes collaboration among community organizations).

Sacks, Swinburn, and Lawrence (2009, p. 76) offer a framework that incorporates three different public health approaches to this problem: "(i) 'upstream' policies that influence either the broad social and economic conditions of society (e.g. taxation, education, social security) or the food and physical activity environments to make healthy eating and physical activity choices easier; (ii) 'midstream' policies are aimed at directly influencing population behaviours; and (iii) 'downstream' policies support health services and clinical interventions."

The following framework was developed by Delgado and Zhou (2008) to implement youth-led health promotion strategies in urban communities, and incorporate active participation of those communities. The framework consists of eight developmental stages, with each stage building upon the previous one. Each of the following stages, in turn, draws upon theory and political considerations.

Stage 1: Building a Team. This stage encompasses all of the elements and activities associated with recruitment, screening, orienting, supporting, and building a health promotion team with complementary skill sets, knowledge, and experiences.

Stage 2: Identifying How Overweight and Obesity Is Thought of As a Community Problem. Local circumstances must dictate how excessive weight is thought about. Is it viewed as a food, environmental, or spatial justice issue (or some combination thereof)? As noted earlier, the particular perspective, or angle, is important in mobilizing a community to action. Are the primary concerns focused on obesity in childhood or obesity in other population groups? This stage sets the marching orders for the intervention.

Stage 3: Identifying Past and Current Efforts. Health promotion must take into account and build upon past and current efforts. This will help shape an intervention by highlighting what has worked or not worked previously.

Stage 4: Planning and Intervention. The first three stages inform how an intervention focused on excessive weight will take shape, including who is the target. This stage can encompass a wide variety of arenas or sites, strategies, and activities, as well as the degree of community participation.

Stage 5: Evaluating. The evaluation stage is complex enough without also contending with community participation. However, this stage must be conceptualized both as gathering data on the success of the intervention and as an opportunity to undertake community capacity enhancement. Thus, training and necessary consultation must be built into this stage.

Stage 6: Reviewing Lessons Learned and Recommendations. The findings from the evaluation will lay the foundation for this stage. Disseminating findings in a way that makes them accessible to communities is an important goal. In addition, establishment of a community public record (document) also becomes important for future generations and efforts in addressing overweight and obesity.

Stage 7: Planning the Next Project. Total elimination or prevention of overweight or obesity is not achievable in the short term. Consequently, building upon efforts takes on importance and leads to the planning of the next project.

Stage 8: Recruiting New Members. Community-based health promotion projects are heavily dependent upon volunteers or paid community staff, and must endeavor to replace members who leave. This stage is also an ideal time to expand and/or include subgroups that are underrepresented. In fact, I would argue that although this stage is specifically devoted to bringing in new members, the process of identifying potential members is ongoing throughout the previous seven stages and is finalized in this stage.

Each of the eight stages brings two important dimensions together: (1) analytical (theory) and (2) interactional (political) considerations. Each stage draws upon theory but must not lose sight of the political aspects of social interventions.

Each stage has a body of theory that can help practitioners shape its conceptualization and implementation. However, this framework does not enjoy the luxury of being viewed strictly from a theoretical perspective; local social and political circumstances must be taken into account (Severance and Zinnah, 2011). For example, hosting a community forum to gather information from the community on how overweight and obesity are taking a toll on residents can work well if the audience consists of residents who are citizens. However, if the residents are primarily undocumented, using a community forum is ill-advised because many undocumented people may fear attending a large gathering in an official public place. Small gatherings, preferably in homes or in trusted establishments (such as houses of worship), might be a better choice.

Health Promotion Interventions

A range of community interventions can lend themselves to addressing overweight- and obesity-related diseases and conditions within an urban context. Health promotion programs focused on excessive weight can be conceptualized in a variety of ways. However, the use of a continuum provides a multifaceted context in which health promotion and its implications for community empowerment and participation can be better understood (table 9.1).

Stage 1 depicts a conventional approach to health promotion programming, with a corresponding embrace of a disease model that places the onus of excessive weight and its consequences on the individual. Each stage that follows takes a progressively more empowering position. Stage 7 illustrates health promotion interventions with the most empowering and community capacity-enhancement perspectives, which are founded upon a social justice approach.

Health promotion interventions can take place in any social arena or setting (Whitehead, 2007). The settings represented in table 9.1 become more community-centered and less traditional with each succeeding stage in decision making. Aranceta, Moreno, Moya, and Anadon (2009, p. S84) note: "Population-based strategies aimed at the primary prevention of obesity should be multifaceted and designed to actively involve stakeholders and other major concerned parties; in addition, multiple settings for implementation should be considered."

Each strategy or practice setting presents certain rewards and unique challenges. Examples related to health intervention at the individual, family, neighborhood, and societal level will follow, illustrating the relationship between intervention and setting, particularly when the community is both a setting for an intervention and part of the solution.

Delgado and Zhou (2008) developed an urban-focused health promotion approach identifying 10 strategies that are particularly relevant in reaching communities of color. I have added two more strategies that can be implemented for a comprehensive approach that considers multiple factors related to food and exercise.

Table 9.1 Decision Making and Health Promotion Programming Dimensions

Health promotion project facet	Stage 1 Service-focused	Stage 2 Development-focused	Stage 3 Leadership-focused	Stage 4 Civic engagement	Stage 5 Engagement with adult staff support	Stage 6 Engagement with adult staff consultation	Stage 7 Community-led
Primary goal	Individual disease/illness treatment	Individual Development	Individual capacity enhancement	Individual capacity enhancement	Individual capacity enhancement	Community capacity enhancement	Community capacity enhancement
Focus of promotion	Individual	Individual	Individual	Individual	Individual	Individual	Community
Process driven	Staff-driven	Staff-driven	Staff-driven	Staff-driven	Consumer-driven with staff support	Consumer-driven with staff support	Consumer- and community-driven
Target of promotion	Individual	Individual	Individual	Individual	Individual	Individual	Community
Setting focus	Agency-based	Agency-based	Agency-based	Agency/community-based	External agency/community-based	External agency/community-based	Community-based
Evaluation	Staff-driven	Staff-driven	Staff-driven	Staff-driven	Staff-driven with youth input	Youth-driven with staff input	Community-driven

1. Media Arts. The development of DVDs that address excessive weight from a culturally competent perspective, for example, can convey important information about healthy eating and physical exercise, in a medium that lends itself to use with individuals, families, and public settings. DVDs are attractive to all age groups, not just youth. Studenski and colleagues (2010) show how they can be effective in increasing physical activity among older adults. The use of local radio and television programs to get across health messages, particularly when supported by the community and involving local celebrities, is another example of media arts programs that are culturally based.

2. Drama. The use of plays to convey information about excessive weight and at the same time involve audiences is still in its infancy. The play *Stages*, developed by the Meerkat Media Collective, is one example of the strategy, in which Puerto Rican youth and older adults come together to tell and interweave their life stories. Storytelling, with its long tradition in many cultures, provides an opportunity for intergenerational participation and can be targeted to particular community subgroups. Neumark-Sztainer and colleagues (2008) report on the effectiveness of an after-school theater program that promoted behavioral change to prevent obesity in children. Jackson, Mullis, and Hughes (2010) see theater as an excellent vehicle for reaching African American adolescents to promote nutrition and exercise.

3. Educational Workshops. Educational workshops can take place in a variety of nontraditional settings (such as homes, community institutions, and open spaces like parks and playgrounds) that are accessible to and respected by communities (Delgado and Zhou, 2008). Drummond and colleagues (2009) describe how educational workshops can be part of an overall strategy targeting child care centers and childhood obesity.

4. Publications. Delgado and Zhou (2008) wrote about the Hyde Square Task Force's Health Careers Ambassadors (Boston) book *Community Health Information Living and Learning,* targeting youth of color on a variety of health concerns, including obesity. These youth put together a book that was culturally competent and targeted members of their community. When publications actively involve the population group targeted, they become more relevant. Note that these publications are only as effective as their distribution plan. In other words, any program should consider how the publications will get into the hands of the target audience.

5. Community Information Campaigns. Community health information programming, often referred to as *social marketing*, lends itself to creative efforts that are culturally competent (Nicheles, 2006). Hyde (2008) sees such programming as an essential part of a comprehensive effort to address obesity. Latinos, for example, tend to rely upon media and their social network (family and friends) to get information on health-related matters (Geana, Kimminau, and Greiner, 2011). Consequently, obesity-related campaigns should tap these sources whenever possible. Reininger and colleagues (2010) recommend community-based participatory research as a means of helping to refine obesity-related messages. Specifically, they discuss an obesity-prevention media campaign for Mexican Americans. Such campaigns can take place in locations that residents frequently use (houses of worship, sporting leagues, local parks and playgrounds, for example) (Campbell et al., 2007; Delgado, 1999).

6. Mentoring of Stakeholders. Focusing on community and institutional stakeholders (individuals with a vested interest and power to influence events and outcomes) offers much promise in addressing excessive weight in communities. Allen (2002) describes how this method can be used to identify and support key community stakeholders, who can then convey effective ways of addressing excessive weight to their communities. Mobach and Catlow (2007) report on the success of a children's healthy activities mentoring program in schools in Australia. Haire-Joshu and colleagues (2010) show the effectiveness of mentoring children on healthy diets and exercise. Smith (2010) presents results from a teen mentors program that also promoted healthy diet and exercise. Kim, Flaskerud, Koniak-Griffin, and Dixon (2005) stress the promise of mentors or lay educators in helping to address health disparities in Latino communities.

7. Visual Arts. The array of visual arts that might be employed includes murals, sculptures, banners, and photographs, among others. The use of *photovoice* (photographing aspects of a community related to a particular theme) has had particular appeal across age groups and in low-income urban communities. In one project, participants were asked to photograph aspects of their community that foster excessive weight, such as junk food advertising and unsafe parks and playgrounds; the results of their research were mounted in an exhibition for the community. Hennessy and colleagues (2010) showed how exhibition could be used to facilitate physical exercise. Photovoice has also proved effective with students in

school cooking and nutrition classes (Everett, Mejia, and Quiroz, 2009). Findholt Michael, Davis, and Brogetti (2010) illustrated its use in developing a better understanding of the roles of diet and exercise in the lives of rural youth.

8. Music and Dance. The importance of music and dance within a cultural context is well understood by those in the helping professions. Both of these performance arts bring deep cultural meaning and serve as a mechanism for celebrations and connectivity for communities. They also have a firm foothold in health program efforts targeting excessive weight. Flores (1995) shows the potential of dance for improving the fitness of African American and Latino adolescents. Epstein, Beecher, Beecher, Graf, and Roemmich (2007) describe the appeal of interactive dance and bicycle games for overweight and typical-weight youth. Murrock and Gary (2010) show the potential of dance in reducing obesity among African American women. Reifsnider, Hargraves, Williams, Cooks, and Hall (2010) discuss the promise of dance for children in a faith-based organization.

9. Gardening. The subject of community gardening will be mentioned only briefly here, since a thorough discussion appears in chapter 11. Gardening is a way to address both the consumption of healthy foods and the need for physical exercise.

10. Health Fairs. The use of fairs to transmit information on overweight and obesity is certainly not new. However, integrating these fairs into community celebratory events, such as parades, provides an opportunity to reach large groups of people in a setting that is culturally meaningful. Cosponsorship of these parades provides an opportunity for organizations that provide weight-focused interventions to publicize their efforts.

11. Social Media. The importance of social media is undeniable, particularly among the younger generation. Hawn (2009) shows how Twitter, Facebook, and other social media are bringing about major changes in how people get health care information. Esparza, Morales-Campos, Mojica, and Parra-Medina (2010) strongly advocate the use of cell phones and social networking as effective means of reaching adolescent Latinas in low-income urban contexts. Orsini (2010) issues a charge to the home health care field to engage social media in reaching out to patients. This means of communication has tremendous potential for addressing overweight and obesity.

12. Social Action Campaigns. Social action campaigns allow communities to come together and demonstrate their concerns about excess weight through collective action. Walls, Peeters, Proietto, and McNeil (2011)

recommend that obesity be addressed through high-level policy and legislation focused on obesogenic environments. Communities can facilitate such action by launching social change efforts that target policymakers.

The twelve health promotion strategies identified above represent only a sampling of the wide range that is available for addressing overweight and obesity in an urban community context. All of the strategies require that communities play active and meaningful roles in conceptualizing and implementing them. The enormity of the challenge necessitates a comprehensive approach on multiple levels. Local circumstances will dictate which of these strategies are most likely to achieve success.

Program Evaluation

Any health promotion intervention must be evaluated in order to gather concrete information about what works and what doesn't work and thereby to inform future efforts. This section will introduce the principles of evaluation and provide an overview of the most notable rewards, challenges, and approaches for evaluation of health interventions focused on overweight and obesity in marginalized communities (Carter et al., 2011; Rains and Ray, 2007; Syme, 2008). For evaluation efforts to succeed, social work must collaborate with other professions (Townshend et al., 2010, p. 19): "While true transdisciplinary research remains a goal rather than an achieved state of our work, we would argue that the very complexity of obesity demands that a more transdisciplinary research is in fact inevitable." Social work, I would argue, needs to be a prominent partner in these efforts.

The emergence and wide acceptance of evidence-based practice has found its way to obesity prevention, which reveals its own set of challenges, particularly in discussing marginalized groups (Waters, 2009). The questions of who determines what constitutes evidence, how best to gather it, and how to analyze it, with implementation as a final goal, are certainly subject to debate. Further, health promotion interventions predicated upon social justice values and utilizing community-based participatory research (CBPR), which is a method that systematically includes community members among those who help to shape and direct a study focused on their groups, also present challenges and rewards.

The principles, framework, and strategies outlined earlier all encourage active community participation, and research and evaluation are no exception. Cargo and Mercer (2008), for example, advocate community-based participatory research for bridging the gap that traditionally exists between research and practice, and Hammond (2009) proposes sophisticated statistical modeling for obesity research as a means of capturing the influence of complex systems on this condition.

This form of research takes on even greater significance when addressing the gap found in marginalized communities. Further, it can be undertaken by a wide variety of population groups. Gob and colleagues (2009), for example, describe one study focused on identifying potential interventions to overcome barriers to adolescents' healthy eating and physical activity. This study identified a series of feasible interventions that are grounded within the operative reality of community youth.

However, as noted by Buchanan, Miller, and Wallerstein (2007, p. 153), ethical challenges arise in conducting this form of research: "Growing use of CBPR raises two new ethical issues that deserve greater public attention: first, the problem of securing informed consent and demonstrating respect for community autonomy when the locus of research shifts from the individual to community level; and second, fair distribution of scarce public resources when practical constraints make the most rigorous research designs for assessing the effects of community interventions virtually impossible."

An entire book could be devoted to the challenges of conducting health promotion research and evaluation on excessive weight and obesity. For purposes of illustration I have selected five rewards/challenges for discussion.

1. The need to do good and do no harm. The motivation to prevent or ameliorate an unhealthy situation provides a powerful incentive for us to enter the social work profession. Seeing individuals and/or communities lose excessive weight and change their image of themselves brings with it great joy. However, as Malterud and Tonstad (2009) warn, it is possible that our practice and research may further stigmatize those who are most vulnerable to being overweight or obese. Consequently, we must endeavor to reach out without engaging in any destructive labeling.

2. Shifting paradigms on research and evaluation. Current research favors medical and surgical solutions to excess weight over health pro-

motion solutions, creating a challenge because of the shifting paradigms about how best to deal with obesity (Yach, Stuckler, and Brownell, 2006). An emphasis on social ecology and health promotion moves us away from a medical model and situates these types of interventions well within a social work mission. Rotegard, Moore, Fagermoen, and Rutland (2010), for example, advance the construct of individual health assets (genes, values, beliefs, and life experiences), which lends itself to a community asset perspective on excessive weight gain. Community assets (such as local houses of worship, culturally based foods, traditions that emphasize healthy eating, and local community gardening) can easily be incorporated into interventions that are community-centered and culturally competent.

3. Expansion of what we mean by community. *Community* is a very complex construct, and expending the effort needed to come up with a definition that gets close to a consensus is time well spent. Social workers as professionals can and should be involved in this process because of the history of community practice that we bring to this discussion.

4. The limitations of community-based health promotion. It certainly is tempting to advocate an approach that will have a positive impact on a problem such as obesity. But it is also important not to oversell any such approach (Merzel and D'Affilitti, 2003). Obesity and excessive weight result from the interplay of numerous factors. A community-based health promotion strategy should not be expected to solve a problem caused by significant social forces, though such a strategy may play an important role in improving the situation,.

5. The complexity of obesity demands multidisciplinary approaches. It is always easy to talk about the virtues of multidisciplinary approaches to health promotion research. The more complex the topic, the more important it is to collaborate. However, collaboration across disciplines, while an appealing idea, is arduous to achieve. Further, when community residents and leaders are included in the effort, collaboration becomes even more challenging because of the need to accept these communities as equal partners.

Social work's long history of working with other disciplines, particularly in the mental health field, has taught us that psychiatry and psychology can be challenging partners as part of treatment teams. The obesity field, I am afraid, will not be any different. Nevertheless, we have no choice but to exert our power through the competencies that we bring and that allow us to function within a community context as part of interagency initiations, coalitions, and task forces.

The expanding field of health promotion, and its potential for achieving significant social change in the lives of this nation's vulnerable communities, certainly presents opportunities for hope and excitement. The use of a socioecological perspective has revealed possibilities for innovative initiatives that facilitate social work's participation in this field. Within the area of overweight and obesity, social work can play an important, if not prominent role. The health promotion perspective, however, takes on significantly greater implications when addressing excessive weight, since any effective intervention must be founded upon a multifaceted set of guiding principles that are empowering, participatory, and embracing of social justice values.

A variety of frameworks, strategies, and settings have been introduced to illustrate the latitude that practitioners have in thinking about how best to address overweight and obesity, taking into account their interests, the organizations they work in, and the circumstances in the local communities. The complexity of the problem means that a concerted effort on the part of social work, and other helping professions, will be necessary in order to achieve any significant degree of success in ameliorating excessive weight and its health and social consequences for marginalized people in this country.

10

Youth-Focused Interventions

There is no nation on earth that can afford to neglect its youth and still hope to play a viable role in a global economy and meet the social and educational needs of its citizens. However, there is no nation that will publicly acknowledge that it systematically and purposefully marginalizes its youth. Rhetoric must be separated from reality and actions, as in the case of the United States.

(DELGADO AND STAPLES, 2008, P. 3)

This chapter provides a glimpse into how youth view overweight and obesity within their group and community, how social justice plays an influential role in shaping youth perspectives on the nature of this crisis, and what needs to be done to achieve positive change. Youth, because of their culture, age, ethnic and racial heritage, and social class, have a unique cultural perspective, which adults (even those from the same cultural background) do not share (Nault, Fitzpatrick, and Howard, 2010).

Interventions targeting youth must be contextualized to take into account the unique position they occupy in their communities and society (Hodge, Jackson, and Vaughn, 2010). Low-income urban youth of color, in addition, must contend with discriminatory forces biased against their age, income, and ethnic/racial backgrounds (Cammarota, 2011; Sutton, 2007). These multiple risks present additional challenges for the development of interventions focusing on excessive weight. Consequently, youth-focused interventions must be contextualized to their communities while maintaining a focus on them as a significant subgroup. Interventions must be age-sensitive if they are to be accepted and successful with this population.

It should be noted that terms such as *children* and *youth* reflect too wide an age range to have significant meaning in the development of interventions. The recent emergence of the descriptor *tweens* represents an attempt to nuance a broader age category.

Sothern, Myers, and Martin (2004) have identified three critical periods for the onset of obesity, each of which has been drawing the attention of scholars and researchers: (1) intrauterine environment or early infancy; (2) 5–7 years of age; and (3) adolescence (Field, 2007b; Nanney, 2007; Stettler, 2007). Each of these periods requires specifically focused assessments and interventions that take into account acculturation levels and gender.

Youth as a Focus

Overweight and obesity are particular issues for youth. Youth are also the primary targets of massive food industry advertising campaigns, and they may not have access to healthy school meals. Further, in many low-income communities, physical education classes have been either reduced or eliminated because of budget shortfalls. Youth of color are at particularly high risk, but unfortunately, very few obesity interventions specifically target them (Wilson, 2009).

Youth, however, bring a unique set of circumstances and rewards to health promotion programs that address overweight and obesity. One is their commitment and ability to socially navigate their own culture. *Culture*, in this instance, encompasses values, music, clothing styles, outlooks, social media preferences, shared experiences, and language. Youth understand what motivates them to engage in certain behaviors, and what it will take for them to change behaviors that are self-destructive, such as unhealthy eating habits and limited physical exercise.

Adults, despite their openness, abilities, and embrace of participatory democratic values, remain outsiders to youth culture, and therefore have an arduous time understanding how weight is perceived and how best to prevent and control overweight and obesity among youth (Aitken, 2001; Boocock and Scott, 2005). Consequently, any effort to address a problem such as overweight and obesity among youth must involve youth in shaping how best to address that problem.

We, as social workers, would strongly question the value of initiatives targeting women that were conceptualized, implemented, and evaluated totally by men. However, we frequently design interventions targeting youth that do not allow the youth themselves to plan, implement, and evaluate them. In many ways, youth are a disenfranchised group. All too often, interventions aimed at youth do not take into account their specific goals, culture, priorities, and preferred methods of engagement in health promotion activities. Those decisions are made by adults.

Youth-led health promotion (Delgado and Zhou, 2008) interventions have at last started to get the recognition they deserve, following much the same path as interventions for older adults have (Delgado, 2009). The potential of youth-led efforts to achieve significant changes in community health, including obesity, was demonstrated in the Humboldt (primarily Latino) community of Chicago (Kelley, Benson, Estrella, and Lugardo, 2009). (The Humboldt Park program will be discussed in more detail in chapter 12.)

Youth-led initiatives also serve as an investment in the future of the community by allocating resources to future adult leaders (Delgado, 2006; Delgado and Humm-Delgado, in press). Youth-led initiatives are a win-win proposition since they address an immediate need or issue—in this case excessive weight—and also help to prepare youth for assuming leadership roles in the future (Delgado and Staples, 2008).

Youth-led initiatives are especially important in marginalized communities. Urban youth, particularly those who have low incomes and are people of color, face even greater challenges in addressing overweight and obesity prevalence in their ranks.

Urban youth of color, however, are not a monolithic entity, which means that even greater attention must be paid to how demographic factors (such as ethnicity/race, gender, level of acculturation, intellectual and physical abilities, and sexual orientation) interact to further increase the likelihood of their being overweight or obese, and how they deal with the health and social consequences of excessive weight (Noguera and Cannella, 2006).

Guthman (2008) suggests that youth in marginalized communities must be encouraged to conceptualize the food justice movement on their own terms and in their own words. Sze (2004), in analyzing Asian American activists, concluded that youth conceptualize environmental justice from a more inclusive perspective and actively seek to integrate issues of oppression, exploitation, and injustice. Further, they bring together public and health concerns; for example, they addressed the plight of farmworkers who have been exposed to pesticides and lead. Kown (2008) found that Asian and Pacific Islander youth activists favored collective action founded upon a critical analysis of their lived experiences with inequalities.

Mair, Sumner, and Rotteau (2008) examine the politics of weight and youth from three vantage points—the food justice movement, the organic farming movement, and the Slow Food Movement—and illustrate how youth are attracted to each of these movements. Each one provides youth with very different options for exercising their rights to participation and shaping the context of food and its impact on their daily lives.

Definition of Youth-Led Health Promotion Intervention

Youth-led health promotion intervention can be defined as intervention that helps youth create lifestyles and living and working conditions that are conducive to health. What makes youth-led health promotion distinctive? Simply stated, it is planned and carried out by youth. This perspective is about understanding power and the social forces that youth must contend with in addressing the role of body weight.

Youth-led interventions, be they health promotion or other types, bring a sociopolitical context that shapes how social problems that impinge on youth are conceptualized (Watts and Guessous, 2006, p. 60): "One alternative to conventional theories of youth psychological and social development is liberation psychology, which is distinguished by its emphasis on human rights and social equity. Exposing social injustice, creating just societies, promoting self-determination and solidarity with others, and ending oppression . . ."

Does this mean that adults cannot be a part of these ventures? No. It means that adults can be partners with youth, but that youth dictate the role that adults assume and the nature of the help that they desire. As Kirshner and Geil (2010, p. 2) put it: "Working class and low-income minority youth rarely have opportunities to participate in settings where consequential decisions are made. . . . The encounters between youth activists and adult community leaders that do occur represent access points for youth, in which young people advocate for their collective interests." Adults can create these opportunities in a purposeful manner and thus maximize youth participation as equal partners and foster youth leadership development.

Youth can join with adults in social activist campaigns to increase the likelihood of success. These types of efforts stress inclusiveness as a value (Kirshner, 2009). Adults, after all, also bring a wealth of resources and experiences, not to mention funding, to this field. Kirshner (2008) illustrates how tensions between adults and youth can be surmounted through facilitation, apprenticeships, and working together. Further, youth-led health promotion is not restricted to their own health and well-being. Goals and concerns can also involve adult family members, neighbors, and residents of their community.

The first case example, later on in this chapter (Healthy Teens on the Move), illustrates how a group of youth were concerned about the well-being of an entire neighborhood that patronized fast-food establishments. Youth-led social change is not just about youth (Fletcher and Vaurus, 2006; Mediratta, 2006); it is also about community (Delgado and Staples, 2008; Hosang, 2006). The case illustrations focus on social action campaigns, although youth-led interventions can encompass all of the strategies for health promotion that have been discussed.

Health Promotion Activities

Youth-led health promotion activities may share much with those of their adult counterparts, but when they do, distinctive elements nevertheless highlight how youth differ from adults in addressing overweight and obesity. For example, youth-led health promotion activities may incorporate music and social media as vehicles for getting information out to other youth.

An emphasis on the "spoken word" among urban youth of color represents another avenue for health promotion messages (Flores-Gonzalez, Rodriguez, and Rodriguez-Muniz, 2006, p. 179): "Spoken word is more part of the performance, and part of the way that your voice is used, the way that your body is used, the emotions in your face. And again, historically, Latinos and blacks have used voice and poetry in forms of communications, and transforming situations into something that's real, and to the youth, poetry and hip-hop, particularly Spoken Word, has a way to deal with reality, has a way to transform, transfer information to one another, and a way to tell stories and just be human."

The Hyde Square Task Force's Health Careers Ambassadors Project in Boston is an example of how low-income adolescents of color (primarily Latino), developed a book on the key health issues confronting adolescents (Delgado and Zhou, 2008). The 25-page book was divided into six sections: (1) what is the health condition; (2) symptoms; (3) causes and risk factors; (4) who is most affected; (5) steps to prevention; and (6) local resources. Excessive weight and the health conditions related to this problem were highlighted in the book. In addition, it used language and photographs that urban adolescents understood, and it was distributed where youth were most likely to find and read it (strategic locations within certain neighborhoods). Youth involved with the Hyde Square Teen Ambassadors Project did have adults helping them as they planned and implemented these activities. However, adults assisted with rather than led the various elements of the project.

Rewards and Challenges

There are numerous rewards associated with youth-led health promotion related to overweight and obesity, and the two case illustrations that follow highlight many of them. Youth are community assets that can be tapped and mobilized in service to other youth as well as to their community-at-large (Kegler et al., 2005). The empowerment that youth experience when they are considered a vital part of their community's well-being is one of the many rewards of a youth-asset perspective and youth-led health promotion. This experience takes on even greater significance when the community they live in is marginalized by the broader society, for through the involvement of the youth, adults begin to see them as contributing members of their community.

Youth participation in the decision-making process is one of the signature elements of this form of health promotion, and it can serve as a model for addressing other health-related concerns. Actions inspired by a social justice orientation, be they focused on health promotion or otherwise, hold much promise for engaging marginalized youth (Cammarota, 2011). On the basis of an in-depth study of youth activists in Calgary, Canada, Lund (2010, p. 23) concluded that they have much to teach adults: "Their insights into student engagement and best practices in enhancing civic engagement of young people can provide valuable findings for practitioners wishing to shape effective social justice strategies and initiatives, and to encourage young people's role as agents working toward social justice in schools and communities."

One of the major challenges in youth-led health promotion (or any other form of social intervention, for that matter) is getting adult professionals to view youth as capable of making decisions (Torre and Fine, 2005). A youth development paradigm shifts conventional deficit-oriented views toward all youth, and marginalized youth in particular. Traditional deficit-oriented views tend to see youth development as apolitical and ignore the ecological environment in which these youth live. Further, such views keep adults in key decision-making roles, relegating youth to participation without the potential of being leaders (Delgado and Staples, 2008; Lewis-Charp, Yu, and Soukamneuth, 2005).

Youth, as the case examples will illustrate, are quite capable of conceptualizing and carrying out social justice campaigns related to food and environment. These efforts can address issues that are common to everyone who lives in the community, regardless of age, since food and environmental justice significantly affect all members of urban communities of color.

Case Examples: Introduction

I have selected two case examples to illustrate youth-led efforts at achieving food justice. Both of them originate in California. Healthy Teens on the Move is a Los Angeles youth-led community-organizing initiative that illustrates the power of youth to create positive change in their communities, and in this case, alter how fast-food restaurants target their community. Youth Envision, in San Francisco, is unique because of its approach to food justice through its support of local business establishments that provide healthy foods at reasonable prices.

Case Example: Healthy Teens on the Move

A Los Angeles case is particularly appropriate in light of how LA's poor and working-class neighborhoods have been targeted by the fast-food industry. The high concentration of people of color in select sectors of this city makes it relatively inexpensive for the fast-food industry to target these groups. Health education efforts focused on encouraging healthy eating habits can be successful only if community members have options to purchase healthy foods. Community members who are educated about the importance of healthy eating but have access only to fast-food restaurants and grocery stores that do not carry fruits, vegetables, whole-grain breads, and non-fat milk, for example, are bound to become frustrated with the situation (Project CAFÉ, 2007). This was particularly true in Los Angeles; after the 1992 riots, supermarkets generally abandoned most low-income neighborhoods in the city, further accentuating a food or grocery gap in these communities (Project CAFÉ, 2007). Consequently, a multi-pronged strategy must educate but also address food justice issues if it is to successfully combat overweight and obesity in low-income neighborhoods.

Healthy Teens on the Move was established by youth in response to their concerns that 60 percent of the adults in their communities were overweight. These youth shared the belief that they could make a difference in their lives, and in those of adults, by encouraging healthier nutrition and physical activity choices in their community.

Healthy Teens on the Move took a multifaceted approach. In 2008, adolescents in Baldwin Park and South Los Angeles instituted a boycott of fast-food establishments that did not include nutritional information on their menus, representing an emerging approach in food justice efforts (Uprising, 2008). (Incidentally, South Los Angeles has one of the highest concentrations of fast-food restaurants in the country, and the city council imposed a one-year moratorium on new fast-food restaurants in the community.) The youth organized a public demonstration and invited community residents (both youth and adults) to join their action. The boycott continued via social media (myspace.com and text messaging) and word-of-mouth campaigns until the fast-food chains finally posted caloric counts on their menu boards.

Healthy Teens on the Move has also offered community education workshops on learning how to read food labels, understanding the importance of portion sizes, what a healthy diet looks like, the consequences of obesity and chronic diseases, fad diets, and the importance of effective physical activity.

One adolescent (Tajah) summed up her concerns regarding fast-food restaurants in their community this way:

> What about the people who become addicted to the food because of all the sugar and fat. There are just so many people who can't seem to stop

eating this poor excuse for food. . . . Every single soul on this Earth is worth fighting for. I work fast food and it's filthy, demeaning, and it's just not a wholesome way to get a meal or to make a living. People are getting sick of paying big $ in exchange for high blood pressure and a big cottage cheese ass. Do not defend McDonald's, as they do not give a woot about your health or your family.

The socioeconomic perspective on fast food expressed by these youth highlights the social justice underpinnings of health promotion and overweight and obesity. Further, the use of social media to pursue the project's goals illustrates the importance of this method for reaching out to youth.

Case Example: Youth Envision

One food justice strategy is to limit the availability of unhealthy food, as in the case of Healthy Teens on the Move. Another perspective, which Youth Envision embraced, seeks to encourage local food establishments, such as grocery and convenience stores, to make healthy food accessible through availability and pricing.

Youth Envision is a youth social activism organization in San Francisco. Its mission statement brings together environmental justice and health, further illustrating how youth of color display a tendency to include health as part of their worldview on social justice (Reed, 2004, p. 2): "The mission . . . is to promote the long-term ecological and human health of Southeastern San Francisco by educating and organizing youth around the principles of environmental justice and urban sustainability."

Youth Envision understood the importance of developing a community intervention based upon local circumstances and definitions of what residents identify as "healthy foods." Youth surveyed 200 community residents about their experiences in accessing healthy foods and found that to be a challenge for most residents. These responses shaped how the Good Neighbor Program was conceptualized.

The Good Neighbor Program targets the city's Bayview Hunters Point community (BVHP), which has approximately 30,000 residents, most of whom are of color and have low incomes. The Good Neighbor Program was funded by a grant from the San Francisco Department of Public Health Tobacco Free Project (Reed, 2004). (The reader may wonder why an anti-tobacco organization was involved. In addition to tobacco companies, Philip Morris owns a number of food companies, including Kraft. Thus, targeting food companies is one way of also targeting tobacco companies.)

The goal of the Youth Envision Good Neighbor project is "to collaborate with local food retail establishments in Bayview Hunters Point neighborhood to promote an environment that encourages healthy living and improves the food resources of all the residents in the community. As such, the replacement of tobacco subsidiary projects with healthy and locally produced food alternatives is essential to the health of the Bayview Hunters Point community" (Reed, 2004, p. 5).

Program participants included high school students residing or attending school in Bayview Hunters Point. They received training in a variety of subject areas related to advocacy. A community capacity enhancement paradigm guided this facet of the program. The time and effort devoted to increasing youth competencies was viewed as an immediate and future investment in the community.

Youth advocates undertook multiple assessments, with each building upon the previous one. The initial assessment selected 11 corner stores along a main avenue in BVHP and assessed the degree to which these stores devoted shelf space to packaged food, alcohol, and cigarettes, all other beverages, produce, meats, and non-food products (Reed, 2004). These items were then color-coded. Youth found that alcohol, tobacco, packaged foods, and non-food products were the most accessible items in the stores, with fresh produce representing only 2 percent of the products sold.

The second assessment specifically focused on the number of Kraft or Nabisco products sold in the stores. Youth found that more than 90 percent of all cookies and almost 80 percent of all cereals and crackers sold were produced by either Kraft or Nabisco (Reed, 2004).

The youth then collaborated with an intern from the University of California, Berkeley, who researched city-sponsored incentive programs for small businesses in San Francisco and found several that could be used to encourage BVHP business owners to participate in the Good Neighbor Program. Merchants, in turn, were interviewed (five out of eleven participated) to get their opinions on their needs and on how to improve access to healthy foods. The grocery stores that were selected to participate had to agree to eliminate all outdoor tobacco and alcohol advertising, stock fresh produce and healthy foods at reasonable prices, comply with laws regulating alcohol and tobacco sales to underage customers, and abide by laws related to loitering, cleanliness, and safety.

Youth Envision developed a brochure describing the program and distributed it to potential participating merchants. Ultimately one establishment was selected to pilot a Good Neighbor store. The program provided this establishment with a $1,000 credit to purchase healthy foods, a selection of energy-efficient upgrades, free advertising in a local newspaper, and in-store promotional activities to attract customers (Reed, 2004). A taste-testing event was held to encourage consumption of fresh produce, and an Earth Day event focused attention on the interplay of food and environmental justice at the community level. Youth advocates also brokered an agreement with the Rainbow Grocery and other food co-ops to provide low-cost and organic products to replace unhealthy products in the Good Neighbor participating stores.

The success of these and other actions resulted in the pilot store's experiencing produce sales totaling 30 percent of the store's retail business, whereas before the store's participation in the program, produce had accounted for only 5 to 10 percent of sales.

Youth Envision's Good Neighbor Program became an active partner in a coalition to foster food justice, but the process did have its share of problems (Reed, 2004, p. 15):

> During the two and one-half year project . . . staff and advocates nurtured relationships with city agencies, community groups, and other nonprofits. . . . Creating a broad coalition had both advantages and disadvantages. On the pro side, the more people involved the better because many different sectors got to know the project and help push it forward. Working collaboratively also provides good support for the project having different city agencies supporting it. On the other hand, agencies operate with different timetables and budget constraints. Because of different funding resources and timeline availability, agencies weren't always able, for example, to provide funding for incentives when they were needed.

Youth Envision also encountered several challenges in seeking to maintain a core group of advocates, among them youth aging out of the program when they graduated from high school and scheduling conflicts with extracurricular activities.

The Youth Envision story of an organization that viewed health from a variety of social justice perspectives illustrates how food and other forms of social justice are united in communities of color (Reed, 2004, p. 15): "Improving community health includes increasing access to healthy foods. Equally as important in the movement to improve community health is the integration of efforts addressing other injustices present in the community, such as violence, environmental justice, racism, and sexism."

These two case illustrations show the potential for youth to constitute a positive force in shaping their environment in relation to fast foods and healthy eating. Both examples also highlight creative ways in which youth address different aspects of food justice. Preventing the expansion of fast-food restaurants within their community, offering nutritional education workshops, and encouraging local businesses to expand their product selection to include healthy food alternatives all represent elements of a comprehensive approach to excessive weight in urban communities of color.

Evaluation Rewards and Challenges

Youth leading and actively participating in health promotion initiatives focused on overweight and obesity, like their adult counterparts, bring a unique set of rewards and challenges to evaluation of these efforts, including their propensity to integrate health with a variety of social activism causes that usually would not include health (Delgado, 2006; Delgado and Zhou, 2008).

The emergence of participatory action research in the field of health has provided a conceptual foundation from which to view youth-led evaluation (Minkler and Wallerstein, 2003) and offers much promise for the field.

Branch and Chester (2009) describe a participatory research study involving adolescents from marginalized backgrounds and propose such studies as a viable means of getting youth from these communities interested in the profession of health research, thereby creating a much-needed "pipeline." Participatory action research embraces community decision making and participation in research, thus facilitating youth involvement and leadership in evaluation.

Nevertheless, youth must contend with a number of challenges in exercising their power to make decisions about evaluation of overweight and obesity interventions. Four key aspects have been identified for discussion, although they do not represent a comprehensive list.

1. Need for Training. Marginalized youth have a strong interest in food environments and research (Nault, Fitzpatrick, and Howard, 2010). They rarely, however, have had an opportunity to participate in conducting research or evaluation projects, although they certainly have been the subject of such endeavors. Consequently, they do not have a rich body of history, experience, and role models for active involvement in research that will have important community implications (Delgado, 2006). Their almost total absence from community research and evaluation efforts has meant that the communities they reside in have suffered from a lack of human capital development.

If youth are to have meaningful roles in evaluating health promotion interventions, adults will need to provide training and field support. Though this may be considered "labor-intensive" or "expensive," it can also be viewed as community capacity enhancement, since the youth will eventually assume adult roles in their respective communities and will make significant contributions to those communities in the meantime (Delgado, 1999; Delgado and Humm-Delgado, in press).

2. Legitimacy of Findings. The results of a youth-led evaluation effort may be viewed as suspect because only "professionals" can assume responsibility for evaluating interventions. A similar argument has been made against adult community residents who do not have the formal research training associated with advanced educational degrees. However, youth face an even greater hurdle because, unlike like their adult counterparts, they simply do not have life experience. This bias stems from an over-reliance on expert educational legitimacy rather than an acknowledgment of experiential expertise legitimacy. Those who think that youth do not have the capacity to undertake research and evaluation studies should be assured that they certainly can do so if they receive the proper training and support (Delgado, 2006).

3. Aging Out. Marginalized youth, if they are lucky, will eventually assume adult roles (even leadership roles) in their communities and in society. The natural aging process brings with it one of the fundamental challenges associated with youth-led interventions: they are bound to age out eventually, thus leaving a vacuum that may be difficult to fill if their exit is not carefully planned for.

However, they can have an opportunity to participate in consultation roles once they become adults (Delgado and Staples, 2008). Aging out is a reality but not necessarily a hindrance, particularly if these newly minted adults have opportunities to serve their communities in other ways, including possibly assisting their youth counterparts.

4. Unique Understanding of Youth Culture. Possession of a knowledge base on youth culture, and the confidence that goes with it, cannot be minimized when launching a youth health promotion initiative. Youth bring a unique understanding of the questions that are salient to their age group and of what activities are likely to succeed in reducing overweight and obesity. Further, they have a profound understanding of how youth use information technology to get information and to communicate with each other. As noted earlier, the food industry has certainly tapped this knowledge in developing marketing strategies that target youth.

Youth also know how to ask questions and how to disseminate findings. Further, when the messages originate from the youth themselves, the likelihood that they will be heard and respected by other youth rises dramatically.

Local knowledge, self-knowledge, and community knowledge can capture information that is not academic in nature but results from life experiences. Youth are the foremost experts on their own needs, lives, and social circumstances. As adults we need to acknowledge this wisdom and tap it as a resource for developing health promotion interventions.

In *Street Science: Community Knowledge and Environmental Health Justice*, Corburn (2005) describes a disconnect between professionals and residents with respect to knowledge of social conditions. This disconnection creates a formidable barrier to the implementation of community-centered interventions. Our abilities as social workers to narrow the gap between these two worlds will go a long way toward enhancing our abilities to actively engage communities in developing health promotion interventions that can successfully prevent and control overweight and obesity, particularly in marginalized urban communities of the country.

Youth represent a vital sector of urban communities and are truly "the future" of these communities. If they are saddled with a host of illnesses and diseases related to excessive weight, their potential to contribute to their families, communities, and the nation itself is seriously compromised.

Youth-led interventions, fortunately, are no longer an alien idea as a means of addressing these issues. Reed (2004, p. 16) sums up the power of youth who participated in Youth Envision:

The project reaffirmed the power of young people as advocates and outreach workers. Their motivation to make positive change in their community is in large part based on their own firsthand experience out of which they can speak personally about the issues. Youth have enormous creative energy in seeing this type of work move forward because it so directly affects their own lives, and those of their families and friends. One of the most challenging aspects for the youth was learning that changing attitudes and actions, and developing strategic ways of sustaining their work take both time and patience.

The role of social work in fostering these efforts is new, and the possibilities for application to many different issues will challenge the profession to develop models that stress participatory democratic principles for all population groups regardless of their age (Delgado and Staples, 2008).

11

Community Garden Interventions

For many participants, urban gardening is a labor of love that combines the best of environmental ethics, social activism, and personal expression. Even when faced with social turmoil, degraded sites, and ambivalent policy makers, urban gardeners maintain a faith that what they do not only helps the individual but strengthens the community.

(LAWSON, 2005, P. 301)

The topic of community gardening has gained currency in the United States over the past 35 to 40 years and particularly in the past decade (Lawson, 2005; Marcias, 2008; Miner, 2010). Community gardens originally sprang up in this country as a response to social and economic crises dating back to the late nineteenth century (Pudup, 2008). Feenstra (1997) argued passionately for the development of local food systems and sustainable communities, and recognized the need for communities not only to consume healthy foods but also to play an active role in their development.

Community gardens represent immense potential for any comprehensive effort at addressing excessive weight, beyond the obvious natural relationship between gardens and a recognition that overcoming overweight and obesity is a worthy goal. That potential goes far beyond the consumption of nutritious food and the achievement of food security, adding a multitude of social, economic, and political benefits that directly affect the prevalence of overweight and obesity in urban communities of color (Baines et al., 2010; Brown, 2010; Hynes and Howe, 2002; Viljoen and Bohn, 2005). When these gardens are planted and cultivated by the community, they achieve a variety of key social, economic, political, educational, and health-related goals (Armstrong, 2000; CDC, 2010c; Lautenschlager and Smith, 2007; Saldivar-Tanaka and Krasny, 2004; Winne, 2005).

A social justice perspective adds an important dimension to community gardens, particularly in its emphasis on community inclusion and participatory democracy (Hansen, 2008). Many practitioners and residents would argue that community gardens encompass many of the key elements of successful community-led interventions to address overweight and obesity of residents.

Prendergast's (2010, p. 1) description of her visit to Vermont Square in East Los Angeles, established right after the Rodney King riots of the early 1990s, provides an excellent context for viewing this garden:

> Upon entering East Los Angeles, the amount of concrete was overwhelming. The cracked asphalt roads bounded by sidewalk shops formed a corridor of fast food restaurants and liquor stores. Nature was non-existent, as nothing about the manufactured world felt organic. Blaring sirens, bustling cars, and wafting fumes overran my senses. Nonetheless it was here that I went to visit Vermont Square: the first garden ever owned by a Los Angeles community. Inside its gates, the calm of the place provided a stark contrast to the blighted neighborhood out of which I had just stepped.

Urban Farming History

The view of the city as a potential source for farming or food production, or even as a farm, may seem odd. The term *urban* is almost invariably associated with negativity. A shift in worldview is needed in order to think of cities as places of vibrant agriculture and food production. Mind you, this shift in thinking is critical for the introduction and viability of farming in the city, and more specifically in marginalized neighborhoods.

Howard's (1946) book *Garden Cities of Tomorrow* argued for dismantling the divide between urban and rural in the conceptualization of farming. Carolyn Steel's more current book, *Hungry City* (2008), argues for viewing the production of food as a means of transforming society economically, socially, and politically. The concentration of food production and consumers in a close geographical area benefits both the producers and the consumers of food by increasing efficiency. Steel's argument parallels the argument put forth in this book that overweight and obesity is a socioeconomic-political issue requiring active consumer involvement, as evidenced through various social justice movements.

The "family farm" has worked its way into American folklore and is very much entrenched in the psyche of the nation. Along with this, an agrarian myth emerged. Yet life on the farm was far from idyllic; it required long hours of hard work and was constantly at the mercy of the elements, not to mention market conditions (Hofstadter, 1964).

Historically, there was no demarcation between urban and rural farming. In fact, many of this nation's cities covered extensive parcels of land, and farming was an integral part of urban life. Eventually, however, farming was relegated to rural sectors of the country because of land availability and cost considerations, resulting in a separation between "urban" and "rural" regions.

The emergence and prominence of cities made city land very costly, and as cities increased in size and population, the farms and the consumers who ate their products grew farther apart (Helm, Stang, and Ireland, 2009). Food production was relegated to geographical areas with large plots of land (farms) that made it economically feasible to produce food. Urban populations, in turn, became more and more removed from the food production process, with big agriculture businesses taking over small farms and increasing farm size in the process. A disconnect and a loss of control over food production resulted. Food became a commodity that could be purchased at a local store, placed alongside paper and plastic products and other items. The symbolic meaning of food was lost (Nordahl, 2009). The sharp divisions of this disconnect, however, have started to blur, as evidenced by the way the green movement has taken hold in many of this nation's urban areas.

Morgan (2009, p. 341), however, contends that urban farming never completely disappeared, and that its alleged disappearance is an "urban myth," although its character and shape certainly changed over the years: "The notion that food production is an exclusively rural activity fails to appreciate the significance of *urban agriculture*, an activity that never disappeared in the hungry cities of the global south and one which is reappearing in the more sustainable cities of the global north." De la Salle and Holland (2010) concur with Morgan's assessment and go on to note that humans can officially be considered an "urban species" and that there is no reason why agriculture cannot be an element in urban life. The prospect of urban areas as potential farmland and as viable and sustainable sources of healthy food production for community residents certainly has its proponents, including this author.

Brown (2002) traces the emergence and prominence of farmers' markets in the United States in the mid-1970s to the passage of the Farmer-to-Consumer Direct Marketing Act of 1976 (P.L. 94–463). More recently, the importance of healthy food, as it is manifested through farmers' markets, has found popularity in many urban communities, including low-income and low-wealth communities. Boston, for example, is considered to have more farmers' markets (27) than any other city in the United States, generating $1.5 million per year, with a 15–20 percent sales increase in 2010 over 2009 (Denison, 2010).

Food production is not the exclusive domain of any particular geographical area, as evidenced by the use of urban areas for farming in other parts of the world over the past 15 years (Mustafa, MacRae, and Mougeot, 1999; Smit, Ratta, and Nasr, 1996).

Alkon (2008) discusses two farmers' markets in San Francisco, one in an affluent community stressing organic foods and wilderness themes and the other in a low-income community of color stressing environmental justice. Both address environmental issues, but from dramatically different perspectives and contexts in terms of race and class. Each market has meaning and value in communities that face very different challenges in daily living and well-being.

It is important to emphasize that urban areas of the country, especially those in coastal regions, have large concentrations of people of color, particularly newcomers (although dispersal patterns are changing and rural and suburban areas are experiencing an influx of newcomers) who have agricultural backgrounds (Delgado, 2011). Consequently, it is not unusual to find urban residents from Asia and Latin America living side by side. They may not share a language and a culture, but they do share a profound love of agriculture (Delgado, 2000).

A number of scholars have specifically addressed the myth that cities cannot engage in farming or food production; when urban areas do participate in those activities, residents who are involved can reap the benefits of access to healthy fruits and vegetables, lower their food budgets, increase physical exercise, and gain more control over their immediate environment (Travaline, 2008). The popularity of the "the city as a farm" characterization captures the urban landscape's potential for food production (Morgan, 2009; Oldham, 2011; Viljoen, 2005).

The emergence of new ways of acquiring locally grown produce in urban areas has introduced some exciting and highly innovative ideas for urban farming. Virtual farming (using artificial light and organic growing materials) and rooftop green gardens, for example, has started to spring up across the country and illustrates how locally grown produce can be economically feasible and preferable to transporting produce across long distances to reach urban markets (Despommier, 2010; Rifkin, 2011).

The environment can also benefit from urban farming, tapping into the environmental and spatial justice movements. Urban farming that makes more efficient use of water supplies, for example, can reduce the need for portable water (Smith, 2008). Converting neglected areas in the community into positive spaces, such as transforming abandoned lots into productive space, is one example of efforts to address spatial justice goals.

Definition of Urban Farming

The phrase *urban garden program* can refer to a wide variety of efforts, such as neighborhood/community gardens, demonstration gardens, relief gardens, children's gardens, entrepreneurial job-training gardens, company gardens, and horticultural gardens, to name just a few. Although these types of gardens have much in common, the goals that they embrace can be significantly different (De la Salle and Holland, 2010). Urban vacant lots, for example, come in many different shapes and sizes, and lend themselves to a great range of urban farming/gardening projects (McMillan, 2008).

Veenhuizen (2006, p. 10) also provides a definition of urban agriculture, or farming, that illustrates its scope: "Urban agriculture can be defined as the growing of plants and the raising of animals for food and other uses within and around cities and towns, and related activities such as the production and delivery of inputs, and the process and marketing of products." The personal consumption or business of urban agriculture brings an added dimension to this form of food production, increasing its potential impact, with public health implications (Brown and Jameson, 2000).

Cities across the country are increasingly turning to agriculture in a variety of forms to help combat food deserts (areas of a community where it is either impossible or nearly impossible to find healthy fruits and vegetables), and Oakland, California, is a prime example of this movement.

McClintock (2008) and Green (2007) provide a detailed accounting and critique of the City of Oakland's effort to generate 30 percent of its food consumption locally through urban agricultural projects as a means of addressing food deserts in the most marginalized areas of the city.

It is critical that social workers and other providers discard a vision of urban farming that essentially transposes rural farms (acreage, equipment, house, barns, etc.) to a city (Baker, 2004; Pudup, 2008). A number of scholars adopted that model during the early and mid-1990s. Hynes's book *A Patch of Eden: America's Inner-City Gardeners* (1995) is arguably the best example of this type of scholarship. Urban farmers must be prepared to occupy relatively small parcels of land and be highly innovative in finding and utilizing space, including rooftops (Armstrong, 2000; Pudup, 2008; Rhoden, 2002). Hotels, for example, have started rooftop gardens for growing fresh vegetables and fruits and keeping bees and, in one case, a dairy goat (Mohn, 2010).

Mougeot (1993), almost two decades ago, proposed a four-step scale for classifying land for urban farming: (1) land unsuitable for building, (2) underdeveloped land, (3) idle public land and bodies of water, and (4) household spaces. Urban farming seeks to put such small parcels of land to productive use, and in the process help to transform the urban landscape in a controlled manner within rather than outside of the community, a key element of any form of social justice.

The productive use of undeveloped or underutilized land in cities, much of which is often owned by various forms of government, converts sites that many would consider to be ugly or detrimental to the health and well-being of community residents into a kind of capital asset (Winne, 2005). The benefits of urban green spaces, in this case community gardens, can go beyond what is typically thought of as nutrition, exercise, and beautification of urban communities (Fam et al., 2008, p. iii):

> Urban vegetation can have a cooling effect. . . . This can reduce building energy consumption by 7–47%. Urban green spaces can have a positive impact on the hydrological characteristics of the highly modified urban catchments. Grasses and treed areas increase water infiltration and slow run-off after rainfall. These areas are also effective at removing significant amounts of pollutants such as phosphorus, lead and nitrogen and fine sediment. Urban parks and golf course[s] can be important "hotspots" of biodiversity in cities.

Lyson, Gillespie, and Hilchey (1995) promoted the use of farmers' markets as a means of fostering bonds of local identity and solidarity, and bridging formal and informal economies. The farm-to-city movement, as characterized by the emergence and prominence of farmers' markets, needs to be examined in a broader perspective to better understand its implications for overweight and obesity reduction in this country (Philpott, 2010, p. 1):

> To enter a farmers' market in a U.S. city in the summer is to experience firsthand the recent revival of small-scale farming. Stand after stand offers a dazzling variety of chemical-free produce, pasture-raised meat and eggs, farmstead cheeses, and more. Yet in a sense, our teeming, bountiful farmers' markets amount to a gloss on a food system that rewards scale and cheapness over all other factors—including quality, nutrition, ecological sustainability, social justice, and a sense of place. While farmers' markets, community-supported agriculture (CSA) programs, and "locavore" restaurants have proliferated over the past decade, they still provide just a tiny portion of the calories consumed by Americans.

The farmers who serve farmers' markets have often been thought of as full-time growers, located outside of urban areas, who on regular schedules bring their products to urban communities for commerce. But it is possible to have farmers' markets that consist of local-urban and part-time farmers who sell the produce grown in community gardens. These businesses, which are often informal, financially benefit the community, since the profits from these ventures can be circulated within the community.

Farmers' markets also provide an important entry point for refugees and immigrants to purchase vegetables that formed a vital part of their diets back home but are difficult to obtain in this country. In 2011, more than two dozen of the farming programs in the United States targeted refugees (Brown, 2011). As more of these and other types of enterprises spring up in urban communities, residents will undoubtedly be attracted to this form of community involvement, which bodes well for the future of this movement and its potential impact on excessive weight within specific communities.

As a further example of the popularity of urban farming, the City of Boston has initiated a plan to convert three city-owned vacant plots (ranging in size from a quarter acre to a half acre) to farmland in the hope of encouraging local efforts to grow fresh fruits and vegetables. Current Boston city law does not allow farming but does allow community gardening; policymakers are seeking to change zoning codes to permit urban agriculture (Irons, 2010). There is hope that other cities will follow Boston's lead, since state and local governments are in a position to foster urban farming on a much larger scale, particularly as plots of land become available through foreclosures.

History of Urban Community Gardening

A brief historical review will illustrate the social and economic forces that led to the urban community garden movement in the United States and explain how this movement can be influential in helping marginalized urban communities address the issue of overweight and obesity. This historical contextualization highlights the interplay of strong economic forces and shortages of food (Hynes and Howe, 2002).

Larson (2005) dates the urban community garden movement in the United States to the 1890s and the birth of three specific programs: (1) the vacant-lot cultivation association, (2) the children's school garden, and (3) the civic garden campaign. The "Victory Gardens" of World War II, however, are often widely credited with reviving national interest in community gardens in urban areas. These gardens were intended to generate food at the local level and thus help the war effort by growing produce to feed the troops.

Scholars trace modern-day efforts at food production through community gardens to the oil crisis of the early 1970s. The cost of food skyrocketed because of rising transportation costs, necessitating local solutions to food shortages. The 1990s witnessed a tremendous growth in this movement (Delgado, 2000), and it has shown no sign of slowing, particularly since a serious economic recession took hold in 2008 that continues to the date of this publication.

Justice and Community Gardens

Urban community gardens can be examined from a multitude of perspectives. A social justice perspective (incorporating food, environmental, and spatial justice) on overweight and obesity suggests that community gardens can be a viable strategy for social work practice, although they rarely appear as part of any social work curricula. However, any urban social worker might encounter community gardens. Invariably, these gardens have been created and maintained without any assistance from social work. That does not mean, however, that there is no role for social work in such ventures (Delgado, 2000).

Open green space and gardening have the potential to address overweight and obesity from multiple viewpoints: the claiming of land for community residents, as places for physical exercise, as conversion of places and spaces that were once open to criminal activity but are now used for productive purposes, and as places for the production of healthy food. How those possibilities get operationalized is very much dictated by local circumstances.

Hung's (2004) description of the East New York Farms Project in Brooklyn highlights how youth interns provide fresh, affordable produce (and thus increase food security), preserve safe public spaces (by converting abandoned, garbage-strewn lots), and create local economic development (through a farmers' market selling produce). Further, Hung sees the value of engaging youth in urban agriculture for immediate and long-term benefits as they transition to adulthood. Youth involved in gardening eventually become adults engaged in gardening. Gardening becomes a community capacity enhancement activity with current and future benefits.

Practitioners in the health promotion field see the potential of community gardens for addressing a multitude of health problems, and are introducing highly innovative projects that combine individual, family, community, and societal goals related to weight and health. This in turn has opened the door for social work and other helping professions to engage in this form of intervention.

Increased physical activity (Catenacci and Wyatt, 2007) and overall healthy lifestyles (Abraham, Sommerhalder, and Abel, 2010; Addy et al., 2004) have been found to be positively associated with gardening. Community gardening has also been found to decrease stress—a key factor that may lead to overeating—and increase positive moods (Sims et al., 2008; Van den Berg and Custers, 2010).

Gardening has been found to increase consumption of fruits and vegetables among adults (Alaimo, Packnett, Miles, and Kruger, 2008) and youth (Allen, Alaimo, Doris, and Perry, 2008; Blair, 2009; McAleese and Rankin, 2007). One study found that having one household member en gaged in community gardening increases the likelihood of that household's consuming fruits and vegetables (1.4 times more than those without a member) and makes it 3.5 times more likely to do so at least 5 times per day (Alaimo, Packett, Miles, and Kruger, 2008). This increase in healthy food consumption, in combination with increased physical activity, effectively combines two essential elements of controlling weight gain.

Community gardens take on even greater importance because of the limited access among low-income Latino and African American communities to supermarkets when compared to white, non-Latino middle-class groups (Mehta and Chang, 2008; Morland, Diez Roux, and Wing, 2006; Powell, Auid, Chaloupka, O'Malley, and Johnston, 2007; Powell, Slater, Mirtcheva, Bao, and Chaloupka, 2007). Further, this field's embrace of a socioecological perspective has also opened the door for the use of social justice values and principles to guide interventions (Martin and Ferris, 2007; Wakefield, Yeudall, Taron, Reynolds, and Skinner, 2007).

Potential Pitfalls of Community Gardening

It certainly would be tempting to extol the virtues of community gardening, including its social justice approach and its positive impact on overweight and obesity outcomes, without qualification. However, the strategy does present some potential drawbacks with respect to overweight and obesity in urban marginalized communities. It is important to include an alternative perspective on urban gardens and urban agriculture, which have sometimes been critiqued as localized efforts to fill in the gaps created by unresponsive government or by neoconservatives and the corporate entities they support (Guthman, 2007; McClintock, 2008).

Pudup (2007) examines the proliferation of gardens in institutional settings that serve marginalized groups, such as schools, hospitals, jails, and other clinical settings. The presence of contaminated soil is a reality in urban communities and that possibility must be checked to avoid the transmission of toxic chemicals such as lead through the produce grown in the gardens (Clark, Bradander, and Erdil, 2006; Finster, Gray, and Binns, 2004).

The following are additional considerations:

1. Urban farming is not for everyone. Although the virtues of urban farming are extolled in this book, agriculture does not enjoy a positive

history with respect to many marginalized groups. The agricultural history of African Americans, for example, dates back to slavery and sharecropping. For some, urban farming revisits this painful period in their family's history. For Latinos, too, urban farming may elicit unpleasant associations with their immediate history of working on "haciendas" or *fincas* (farms) where they toiled for subsistence wages. Coming to the United States was an effort to leave that past behind, and working on an urban farm may be frowned upon.

Carter (2010, p. x) makes a similar observation on the significance of farming in marginalized communities of color: "Some Americans associate working the land with slavery. A great tide of African Americans migrated from the South to the industrial cities of the North to escape the land and everything associated with it. . . . The land was something you left behind. In the minds of many of our relatives and ancestors, the more distant you were from the past, the better." Thus it might well be unreasonable to expect African American and Latino communities to quickly embrace urban agriculture.

2. Time and energy for farming. The prospect of working in a community garden after working a day job, particularly for those with more than one day job, is anything but romantic and energizing. Gardening or farming is a labor-intensive process, as evidenced by the mass exodus from farms over the past several decades. Further, it invariably means working outdoors, sometimes during less than ideal conditions for those who are not lucky enough to live in a temperate climate.

Consequently, a careful assessment of a community's residents is essential before proposing and supporting an urban garden program. In local schools, however, gardening is both feasible and advisable, and schools should be encouraged and supported in pursuing it. Eventually, the parents and guardians of the students may be inspired to undertake gardening themselves.

3. Patience is a virtue if you can afford to wait. Farming or gardening is a process that unfolds over an extended period of time. Although I do advocate the use of community gardening to create a sense of community and enhance community capacity (Delgado, 2000), it requires long-term planning, preparing the land, planting, and harvesting. This gardening cycle may unfold over many months depending upon local circumstances. Gardening in the winter, for example, in urban regions that experience harsh weather at that time of year, does not help put food on the table

during those months. Thus, seasonal variations and alternatives to gardening are needed in order to take weather into account.

The off season is an excellent time to celebrate, plan, and explore potential sites that can be converted into gardens. Consequently, gardening can best be thought of as a year-round activity with slow periods. Fund-raising, for example, can be done during the slow periods. Urban gardening, like its rural counterpart, always has something that needs to be done.

4. Can we afford to devote precious land to farming? Urban land is very expensive when compared to rural land. Further, large vacant lots, which lend themselves to large urban gardens, could also be used to develop affordable or low-income housing, or to encourage economic development as stores or factories (Lawson, 2005, p. 299):

> Today most gardens make opportunistic use of vacant or underutilized land, but changes in the economy or local conditions may mean that, sooner or later, the site becomes valuable for other development. The battle to protect community gardens in New York City in the late 1990s highlights the fragility of unprotected gardens in cities that experience development booms. No one wants to see the product of hours of hard work leveled by a bulldozer.

Thus, tensions will emerge in determining how best to use large or even relatively small parcels of land for the betterment of the community and who is the ultimate judge of this decision (Nordahl, 2009).

Those who favor open spaces, gardens, and greenery will find themselves on the opposite side from those residents who favor increased affordable housing, for example. Not everyone in a community will support using large parcels of land for farming when there are significant numbers of community residents who live in substandard housing or are homeless. Competing goals and values are to be expected. Furthermore, urban centers generally include plots of available land that are owned by various governmental entities. The government's goals for maximizing tax revenues may be at odds with those of community residents who favor agricultural use. However, it is possible to construct a win-win situation in which all sectors of a community benefit.

Case Examples: Introduction

Community gardens facilitate comprehensive approaches that successfully allow health promotion to be conceptualized along a range of dimensions, including social justice–inspired change. Such efforts increase food access through participatory democracy principles that not only result in better nutrition and provide avenues for physical activity but also empower participants.

Larson (2005) conceptualizes urban gardens as community resources or assets that can address community developmental needs and engage in interest-based activities that foster collaboration across many spheres. However, community urban gardens must not be seen as a "panacea" for all community problems. They may be a part of local solutions, but they are not the sole solution to overweight and obesity.

The first case example originated in the South Bronx, New York City (birthplace of the author), and illustrates the role of community gardens and their potential contributions when they are part of a community-based coalition. Community gardens can result in many different types of collaboration (Arrom, 2006b). This example shows how community gardens can meet a range of community needs. The second example illustrates how communities can reclaim vacant land and convert it to community-dictated purposes such as gardening and physical exercise.

Case Example: La Familia Verde (The Green Family)

La Familia Verde was selected because it represents a community gardening coalition in several neighborhoods of the Bronx, New York City, and presages a forthcoming discussion of community-based interventions. Founded in 1998, La Familia Verde embraces a wide range of projects and gardens that are possibilities for sustainable food practice in an urban community.

Karen Washington, the primary creator of La Familia Verde, provides a brief historical overview of the organization: "La Familia Verde means The Green Family. It was formed back in 1998 and it was a result of the crisis that was going through the city regarding vacant lots and open space. Some of the gardens in this area were threatened and had no where to turn. And everyone knows that where there is unity, there's strength."

La Familia Verde's primary mission is to "sustain the environment and culture of our neighborhood through education, community service, and horticulture." This mission was borne out during a turbulent time in New York City's history regarding community control over gardens:

> La Familia Verde was formed due to the City's quest to auction off over 100 community gardens. It was time to take a stand. The "community" part of gardening had to take center stage. As we gathered gardeners' support throughout the City, we also received support from the community at large. As the community saw us fight for garden preservation, social issues in our own community started to surface. Community gardeners started addressing issues such as affordable housing, school overcrowding, safe streets, unemployment, and immigration.

La Familia Verde established key alliances with several community groups and has a distinguished history of fostering activism and community pride along with sustainable food practices. Its mission is multifaceted and includes creating and sustaining the local environment and culture, and it boasts five community gardens, a community-run farmers' market that sells produce from the gardens, cooking demonstrations, and a community-supported agriculture (CSA) system. The program serves as a prime example of the potential of a multifaceted approach to community gardening and its implications for empowering impoverished urban neighborhoods with affordable food and collective community pride.

As of 2011, there were eight active community gardens. La Familia Verde has also reached out to schools, since the gardens can function as an environmental resource for educational instruction. The organization also works closely with the police department in an effort to reduce crime in the neighborhood. La Familia Verde's farmers' market has increased community access to fresh vegetables and fruits. Every two weeks cooking demonstrations are offered, which include free samples, with a focus on fresh produce and how it can be cooked in a simple but culturally affirming manner. Workshop participants receive a two-dollar Health Bucks coupon that can go toward purchase of fresh produce at the farmers' market.

La Familia Verde has a history of partnering with community organizing groups (such as the Croton Community Coalition and the Northwest Bronx Community and Clergy Coalition) to address social justice issues. It has also collaborated with other local environmental organizations (such as Bronx Green-Up, Green Guerillas, and Operation Green Thumb) to attract valuable resources to maintain their gardens. In the fall, La Familia Verde sponsors a harvest fair in collaboration with the Parks Department's GreenThumb, Just Food, and the New York Botanical Garden. This fair attracts community gardeners from throughout New York City for a competition and also features competitive athletic events.

La Familia Verde has also undertaken highly innovative projects such as Trees for Life and Unity, a September 11 memorial consisting of trees:

> The planting of memorial trees serve[s] to remember the victims of the tragedy and will provide community gardens with the trees they need but cannot afford. La Familia Verde hopes that these trees will also work to address their priority areas of health benefit in an area with a disproportionately high asthma rate. Moreover . . . La Familia Verde uses plantings as a chance to promote positive inter-racial, cultural, and lingual relations—an important end in an extremely international area with many recent immigrants from Africa, Mexico, and the Caribbean.

As of 2011, 40 trees had been planted and more were planned. This project was undertaken in collaboration with Green Guerillas.

As is evident, La Familia Verde excellently illustrates the close relationships between justice, health promotion, and social change.

Case Example: Santa Ana Community Park and Center

The Santa Ana Community Park and Center does a wonderful job of tying together various approaches by showing how communities can convert and develop green spaces to serve multiple purposes, including growing food and providing space for recreation and physical exercise. Urban areas have historically had sizable amounts of vacant land in their midst that could serve these important functions but are generally controlled by governmental entities. Getting governmental authorities to turn these properties over to local communities invariably requires mounting social action campaigns that stress the injustices being perpetrated on low-income communities, whose residents often are people of color.

Santa Ana is located in Orange County, California, one of the wealthiest counties in the United States, a county where 32,000 acres have been established for parkland and open space. Unfortunately, none of this land is located in Santa Ana, a city where 34.8 percent of children are classified as obese, the highest percentage in California's 10 largest cities (Latino Coalition for a Healthy California, 2006).

The injustice associated with the limited access to green space is not uncommon in low-income urban communities of color such as Santa Ana. In the words of America Bracho, founder of Latino Health Access:

> I have to confess, when I see vacant lots . . . I see injustice. If we are invisible to the people that allocate money, if we are invisible to the people that do planning, if we are invisible to the people that have the resources, there is something wrong with that picture. If you can make the decision, as a political representative, or as the leader of an institution, you can make the decision of putting a park in a place and liquor stores in another place and you put the liquor stores in my neighborhood, and the parks in the other neighborhood, there is something very wrong with that.

Latino residents of Santa Ana staged a rally to convert a half-acre empty lot into a community park and center. In collaboration with Latino Health Access, a community-based organization, "residents were able to garner the support of local civil engineers, architects, and contractors who agreed to volunteer their time and develop the park in addition to a jogging trail, exercise stations, and a community center" (Latino Coalition for a Healthy California, 2006, p. 8).

A small group of mothers also created flyers, knocked on doors, and recruited other parents to lobby city officials to approve their plans and grant ownership of the park to Latino Health Access. The park's creation was community-driven and residents worked to have it become community-owned; this park and community center not only helped to promote physical activity and healthier eating, but also empowered community residents to take control of their community, an important goal in social justice campaigns addressing obesogenic environments. In October 2008, the City Council of Santa Ana, along with the city's planning division, completed the Latino Health Access Park and Community Center's site plan review and initiated a $4 million capital campaign.

The Park Resident Advisory Committee was established to aid in the design and development of the park. Residents sit on the eight-person Community Park Advisory Board and serve as community advocates for open space. This park is intended to be the site for a wide range of programs and activities that specifically address family health and wellness concerns.

Dr. America Bracho stated what the park represents to the community (Latino Health Access, 2009, p. 1):

> This land is more than dirt. This land is the dream of seven years for our community to have a place where our children can play. For this project to get this far, we have had to do a lot of asking. But, it doesn't matter, I'm not ashamed to ask. And no one should feel ashamed of asking and fighting. What we should feel ashamed about is not participating in providing our families a better life. Because if we don't do it, no one is going to. This park is here because we chose to participate.

In November 2010, the community broke ground on the park. Planning and fund-raising are still ongoing as this book goes to press. The promise of this community-inspired and -directed effort illustrates the empowerment that can result when a community comes together to claim open land within its borders. The importance of a social justice perspective is inspiring, and illustrates how the community, in collaboration with a well-respected community agency, found the voice and the power to take control of its environment. Vacant plots of land should never be allowed to exist in low-income urban communities that are in desperate need of places for recreation and the growing of fresh produce.

Evaluation Rewards and Challenges

Evaluating the impact of community gardens and open plots of land is facilitated because of the very physical nature of this form of capital. Unfortunately, there are not many published evaluation studies of community gardens, despite the popularity of this method of urban farming (Alaimo et al., 2008; McCormack, Laska, Larson, and Story, 2010), and methodological challenges abound (Twiss et al., 2003). Thus, measuring the benefits can be quite challenging, particularly if one takes a comprehensive approach that seeks to measure the amount of healthy foods that have replaced unhealthy foods in diets, financial savings from gardens, the extent of physical exercise before and after commencing gardening, real estate price changes in property surrounding gardens, and the social change efforts that have been initiated and can be traced back to community gardens. Wills, Chinemana, and Rudolph (2010), for example, found that one of the outcomes of a community garden in Johannesburg, South Africa, was the development of trust between various organizational entities working together on the garden. In essence, what may appear to be simple and straightforward is anything but that.

Baines and colleagues (2010, p. 13) note that there is no one model for the ideal garden but there are several themes that are common to successful gardens: "All gardens must start with thoughtful planning through reflective conversations of all interested parties and the development of a few key leaders to take responsibility for the future of the garden. Once leaders and participants have been identified, the garden's size and structure must be determined based on availability of land, number of interested parties, and resources of community partners." The decision-making process plays a critical role in determining the ultimate success of the endeavor.

The emergence of GIS technology now allows us to accurately measure proximity to parks (Mcintyre, Macdonald, and Ellaway, 2008). This method allows for actual measurement and perceived distance to parks, as well as other green space, and therefore calculation of population-based interventions. Physical proximity to parks and gardens, however, is quite complex, and must take into account dimensions related to psychological access as well, such as feelings of safety, welcoming space, and lack of significant geographical barriers, which should be included in any comprehensive measure of physical access (Powarka, Kaczyski, and Flack, 2008).

Nevertheless, evaluation of community gardening and overweight and obesity can be accomplished when methodology seeks to actively include community residents in all facets of the undertaking. Professional input and partnerships will be necessary if the methodology is to be successful and if the final results are to be accepted both within and outside the community. Fortunately, more and more efforts at instituting evaluation of community gardens and public green spaces are being reported in the literature.

The greening of urban centers and the food derived from gardening are very much alive and quite diverse. Local conditions wield profound influence on how local communities embrace this movement (Tavernise, 2011c), and community gardens are but one manifestation of it.

The social justice implications of this movement, too, can play out in a variety of ways, such as increases in nutritious food consumption and physical exercise, as well as many forms of capital (human, economic, social, cultural, and political). Low-income/low-wealth urban communities can tap the momentum of the urban greening movement to benefit all sectors of the community, but particularly all age groups. Community gardens represent only one element of a potential multifaceted, community-based approach to excessive weight.

12

Community-Based Food Initiatives

The U.S. economic crisis provides a unique opportunity to examine questions of fundamental importance to public health. Does society wish to produce vast amounts of low-quality food, neglect the social infrastructure to support physical activity, and sustain the inevitable economic and social harms of obesity-related diseases? Or will this opportunity to align economic and social policies with the interest of public health be seized by implementing a comprehensive, national obesity strategy? Failure to act now could ultimately cost society much more than even the sub-prime mortgage crisis.
(LUDWIG AND POLLACK, 2009, P. 535)

The economic crisis that confronts this nation in 2012 can be used as an excuse to avoid doing anything of substance about overweight and obesity. However, as any good social worker would know, a crisis is an excellent time to do things that are bold.

Confronting the problem of excessive weight in general, and its increased prevalence in certain communities in particular, requires a bold vision and the active involvement of communities (Huberty et al., 2010), which can play an influential role in devising the needed interventions. The implementation of participatory democratic principles, which has long been typical of social work, can benefit communities in ways that go far beyond simply reducing excessive weight.

The role of community in shaping interventions to address overweight and obesity, founded in social justice principles, characterizes the health promotion interventions advocated throughout this book. They emphasize alternatives to conventional (medical- and deficit-oriented) approaches in urban marginalized communities (Day, 2006). Community becomes not just the focus of interventions but also the source, process, target, and setting for interventions (Kegler, Rigler, and Honeycutt, 2010).

This perspective runs counter to most forms of intervention, which stress professional control of the entire process, with minimal, if not token, community participation; the community is viewed as the target of change rather than as an active decision-making player in the process, a view that fails to take into account the complexity of communities.

Brownell (2007, p. 124) sees tremendous value in consumer-led efforts manifested through community activism:

> In the United States, the ingenuity in addressing obesity is occurring at the grass roots. Changes beginning at the grass roots can grow into a powerful social movement, one that builds in size and momentum and then forces the systemic change necessary for national action. The relatively limited and weak—in a structural sense—actions of the U.S. government cause America—a major contributor [to] the problem on a global scale—to lag behind many other nations or regions in progress on the obesity epidemic.

Hess (2009) provides a highly detailed account of how local movements can counteract global trends that disempower communities.

Community-initiated interventions predicated on social justice principles bring to the forefront goals of empowerment, participatory democracy, and indigenous leadership development, in addition to specifically addressing overweight and obesity among residents. Though there are many types of community-led social justice interventions, those centered on food justice are a frequently encountered example. Food justice represents an all-encompassing concept that shapes community interventions, including those that are focused on health promotion (Griffith, 2003). Health-promotion-focused food justice community interventions generally aim to increase access to healthy food and/or decrease availability of unhealthy fast foods or junk foods in low-income communities of color.

As noted earlier, such interventions include public education campaigns to raise awareness in the community, efforts at controlling food production and availability, and social action efforts to alter practices and policies (at the local and state levels). Thus the different levels of focus satisfy one of the critical criteria for health promotion. Flores (2008, p. 370), however, warns us about how these campaigns get framed:

> Finally, and perhaps most importantly, researchers and advocates for health and the environment must use more effective frames and messages that resonate with Latino and non-Latino audiences alike. Even the best scientific evidence doesn't necessarily translate into public policy,

much less behavior change. Getting others to believe and act on creating healthier environments starts with building relationships and strengthening communications across cultures and disciplines. Latino communities are an essential part of the solution.

This chapter discusses how social justice, health promotion, and community action can combine forces to help communities address issues of overweight and obesity. It begins with describing community-led versus community-participation initiatives and then moves on to examine leadership development, the use of coalitions/task forces, and the importance of evaluation. These aspects of the issue have been featured because they are particularly attractive for meaningful community involvement in excessive weight interventions, and social workers are well versed in these topics.

Two in-depth case studies illustrate how key theoretical concepts can be applied in an urban community program that addresses overweight and obesity among people of color, particularly youth. These urban initiatives help to show the broad reach of health promotion when ecological and justice perspectives guide the intervention but also acknowledge the challenges that are involved.

Community-Led Initiatives Versus Community Participation Initiatives

The concept of community is one that every helping profession is well aware of and embraces to one degree or another as an important factor in service delivery (Delgado and Humm-Delgado, in press). How a community is conceptualized (since communities are never monolithic in structure) will wield considerable influence on initiatives that focus on excessive weight.

There are major differences between "community-led" and "community-participation" initiatives. The latter term signifies only "participation" and does not differentiate between the level of participation and decision-making power. Thus, when the term *community participation* is used, it invariably refers to community membership with minimal sharing of power between institutions and the community they serve.

Community-led initiatives signifies that the decision-making power rests with the community, through its leaders and representatives from community-based institutions and organizations. These individuals are accountable to their community rather than to any governmental or regulatory authority.

The term *community-based* can have a wide range of meanings. This type of intervention may be based in the community and take a group-focused rather than an individual-focused approach. *Community-based* can also mean that communities are the target of an intervention and residents are playing prominent (decision-making) roles in carrying out the intervention. Community, consequently, can be a target of, a vehicle for, or even a philosophical stance in guiding overweight and obesity interventions.

Clarity about how these terms are used is important, since they wield considerable influence on the degree and nature of resident participation in an overweight- or obesity-focused initiative. I prefer community-led initiatives because they encompass the democratic participatory principles that are familiar to the social work profession and they place decision-making power in the hands of residents and indigenous leaders. However, in communities with minimal or no history of active participation and no previous cultivation of indigenous leadership, community-led interventions may not be immediately possible. In such a case, the interventions chosen must ultimately build toward community leadership, with all of its rewards and challenges, with community capacity enhancement as a central goal.

Community-Led Efforts

Efforts at reversing America's 30-year trend of weight gain (which is predicted to continue well into the future) will require a long-term commitment and comprehensive initiatives with communities at their center. Community-led initiatives are certainly not new; however, it has been only in the last five to seven years that they have received the recognition that they deserve for addressing excessive weight within a community context. In many ways, the United States has lagged behind other countries in this form of intervention. Peters, Ellis, Goyder, and Blank (2005), for example, note that community-led efforts to address overweight and obesity in England can be traced back to the end of the twentieth century (1998).

Findings from this initiative, as well as others, reinforce the central premise of this book by arguing that community involvement is critical to the success of interventions that address health inequalities. Increased involvement of the community in decision making results in greater impact for the intervention. For example, the Massachusetts Public Health Association (Friedman, 2005) published the book *Community Action to Change School Food Policy: An Organizing Kit,* which specifically helps residents to use social action to change policies that encourage unhealthy food consumption in local school districts, and typifies a social justice approach to overweight and obesity.

Community-led efforts at addressing overweight and obesity are also more likely to be culturally competent. Murrock and Gary (2010), for example, describe the success of using dance to increase physical activity among African American women. These dances were held at two local African American churches and were led by a community member. James and colleagues (2008) report on the success of getting Latina mothers and daughters (third through sixth grades) to participate in nutrition and exercise activities such as salsa and samba dancing. Warren and colleagues (2009) report on two health promotion nutrition-exercise projects based in Raleigh, North Carolina, that actively involved church volunteers.

Making interventions culturally competent is never an easy goal but it is an essential one. As noted earlier, culture is never static. In the case of newcomers to this country, for example, cultural values, beliefs, and traditions become a moving target, depending upon the age of family members, gender, and the age at which they arrived in this country. Consequently, families as a unit do not acculturate at the same pace.

Early identification of chronic diseases and community involvement in meaningful community research is a critical step in helping to address health disparities in marginalized communities, and can also allow for community capacity enhancement in the process. Capacity enhancement must always be integrated into any community effort that addresses overweight and obesity. The degree to which this goal can be achieved depends upon the professionals involved and the expressed desires of the residents of the community.

Leadership Development

Social-justice-inspired efforts at enhancing community capacity to address overweight and obesity and other social and health concerns must develop and support indigenous community leadership if they are to be sustained over time. The crisis of overweight and obesity in marginalized communities will not be solved quickly. Consequently, community-led efforts and community-based initiatives must actively seek to develop a cadre of community leaders with the requisite knowledge and competencies to address the chronic illnesses associated with overweight and obesity.

Even community-based interventions that are not community-led can enhance community capacity through leadership development. The process of identifying and developing leaders must include active efforts to empower under-represented groups such as youth, older adults, women, the GLBT community, and people with disabilities. Involvement of these disenfranchised groups in community efforts may pose a challenge, since the same oppressive forces that marginalize these groups in the broader society may also operate within communities.

San Diego's Mid-City CAN Coalition illustrates the potential and the unique contributions of Latino community residents as leaders and participants. The establishment of the Latinos y Latinas en Acción (LLEA), and the hiring of a Latino community organizer from Mid-City, played an instrumental role in the success of the coalition, but such efforts are labor-intensive (O'Neill, Williams, and Reznik, 2008, p. S40): "As the literature suggests, effective community mobilizing can lead to genuine, sustained leadership from partnership with residents, but the process must begin with small steps and often takes years to develop. The community development process takes time to mature. Many funding agencies and community leaders demand immediate results, and tend to prefer flashy, 'photo-op' events that seem to demonstrate impact."

Local leadership development has to be a central goal of any excessive-weight initiative targeting urban low-income communities of color. Assessment of the skills acquired by community members in these coalitions is a necessary part of any evaluation of health initiatives (Kegler, Norton, and Aronson, 2007). Local leadership, too, must not be restricted to any particular subgroup (adults, for example); rather it should endeavor to broaden the community leadership pool.

Sometimes obesity initiatives seek to tap the existing leadership within a community because that approach is relatively easy to implement. However, these individuals may not be the best leaders for an overweight and obesity campaign. Although it is tempting to assume that existing leaders are able to cut across issues and population groups, this is often far from true. We would be hard-pressed to find an older adult who is considered a leader among youth, or a man who is considered a leader on women's issues, or a youth who is a leader on adult issues. The legitimacy that comes with being a leader is not boundless, and it is very much determined by the individual's characteristics and group membership. Thus, hard work will be required to identify and nurture new leaders who are best equipped to address the topic of excessive weight.

Coalitions

The problem of overweight and obesity is too great to be addressed by any one entity, regardless of that entity's size and resources. Further, even a collaboration among various entities, prominently including the community of interest, will have to be prepared to sustain initiated efforts over an extended period of time. These challenges can best be addressed through the establishment of broad-based and inclusive coalitions. The CDC has identified community coalitions or partnerships as an effective strategy for undertaking obesity prevention initiatives (Khan et al., 2009).

The potential of such community structures is gaining attention in efforts to address overweight and obesity (Pothukuchi, Joseph, Burton, and Fisher, 2002, p. 3): "As advocates seek to address a range of interconnected food system problems, they may find that building partnerships and coordinating efforts is essential to developing effective and lasting solutions." Garcia and Fenwick (2008) advocate a multifaceted approach (strategic campaigns, coalition building, research, use of media, and policy and legal advocacy within and outside courts) as a means of undertaking school-based social-justice-inspired initiatives to address overweight and obesity in marginalized urban communities.

Community coalitions can become a vehicle for making communities central in the planning, implementation, and evaluation of an intervention. The most promising community interventions have coalitions prominently featured. Thus, we pay special attention to the role and function of coalitions and task forces, although these vehicles are certainly not the only viable option in developing community-based overweight and obesity interventions.

The University of Michigan's Center for Managing Chronic Disease (2007) strongly recommends the creation of community coalitions to address the multifaceted aspects of overweight and obesity. The University of Pennsylvania's Netter Center for Community Partnerships, through its Agatson Urban Nutrition Initiative, has sponsored coalition development, youth-led organizing, peer education, internships, and school gardens. These two programs only touch upon the possibilities of coalitions' coming together to sponsor community interventions focused on reducing and preventing overweight and obesity. Lewis and colleagues (2011) add further credence to the idea. The African Americans Building a Legacy of Health Coalition successfully addressed food deserts in South Los Angeles.

Coalitions can be quite effective even when their goals are focused on just one food item or a very specific population group, such as children. Golub, Charlop, Groisman-Perelstein, Ruddock, and Calman (2011) report on the success of a New York City coalition effort in 2006 that targeted making low-fat milk available in 1,579 schools, serving 120 million containers of milk per year. The coalition was also successful in reducing the availability of sweetened milk, as a means of improving nutrition in the city's schools.

These types of coalitions provide a foundation, or common ground, from which "creative" solutions can emerge that take into account local circumstances. In addition, such coalitions facilitate the marshaling of resources and political will to address what appears on the surface to be an intractable social and health problem. Placing overweight and obesity within a community context helps to ensure that local stakeholders and residents play a significant role in the creation of solutions (University of Michigan, 2007, p. 9): "The inclusive approach . . . can foster solutions developed in concert with those who are most intimately connected to a problem and can therefore enhance the chances that solutions will be accepted and used."

Community coalitions have the potential for addressing overweight and obesity through a variety of strategies on the individual, family, community, and social policy levels, as well as for building the community and organizational capacity to address other local social and health needs. They become an avenue through which community-based efforts can be initiated and monitored, and they can serve as a springboard to other topics related to health disparities.

Coalitions can take many different shapes. Here we focus on those that have local residents and stakeholders as critical partners, with professionals assisting residents rather than "driving" the coalition. The size and membership are dictated by the indigenous leadership as a means of ensuring that the outcomes of interventions meet the needs of the community. Coalitions can be structured with flexible subcommittees whose membership can be tailored to address specific activities and tasks that emerge over the course of an intervention.

Food policy councils are another version of a government-private coalition or task force. Since their beginning in 1982 (the first in the nation was located in Knoxville, Tennessee), food policy councils have attempted to centralize community food-related topics to avoid gaps, duplication, and counter-actions by government. They generally seek to address all or a combination of the following food-related goals (Harper, Shattuck, Holt-Giménez, Alkon, and Lambrick, 2009, p. 2): "1. To serve as forums for discussing food issues. 2. To foster coordination between sectors in the food system. 3. To evaluate and influence policy. 4. To launch or support programs and services that address local needs." These goals can easily be cast as a health promotion strategy.

Needless to say, social workers should be an essential part of these coalitions. Unfortunately, that is not always the case. The Chicago Food System Collaborative, for example, which addressed youth of color in Chicago's low-income communities, involved eight different professions, but social work was not one of them (Suarez-Balcazar et al., 2006). This omission seriously limits our potential to achieve significant social change on a health matter of extreme importance in the lives of those we hope to help.

Case Examples: Introduction

Selecting case examples for this chapter was challenging, not because of an absence of examples but rather because there were a great many good candidates. Pothukuchi and colleagues (2002, p. 3) capture the array of community-based initiatives that are possible in response to an assessment of local needs and assets: "In communities across the nation, advocates and organizations are working hard to develop solutions to food system problems and create innovative models that meet community needs. They are providing food to the hungry, creating community food businesses, organizing food policy councils, developing community gardens in inner-city neighborhoods, and linking consumers with local farmers through farmers' markets, along with many other initiatives."

The case examples presented in chapters 10 and 11 provide a rich and detailed illustration of how and why communities must be a part of health promotion initiatives targeting overweight and obesity. The two examples for this chapter, however, are distinct in that they signify a shift toward practice involving a collection of people and organizations.

Case Example: Chicago's Community Organizing for Obesity Prevention (CO-OP)

The case of Chicago's Community Organizing for Obesity Prevention (CO-OP) brings together various themes raised earlier (Becker, Longjohn, and Christoffel, 2008; Margellos-Anast, Shah, and Whitman, 2008; Suarez-Balcazar et al., 2006). It illustrates a variety of community-led efforts and shows the potential for different entities (organizations and residents) to form coalitions or consortiums to obtain funding (through the Robert Woods Johnson Foundation) for overweight and obesity initiatives, which are tailored to meet local community characteristics and circumstances.

The Humboldt Park dimension of the CO-OP initiative (CO-OP HP) seeks to localize projects at the community level. This effort was sponsored by a consortium of organizations and community activists, and housed at the Center on Obesity Management and Prevention of Chicago's Memorial Research Center. Chicago's Humboldt Park community consists primarily of Latino and African American residents, and was targeted for a variety of community-led initiatives such as organizing a farmers' market, recruiting volunteers to distribute fresh produce through the Greater Chicago Food Bank Depository, organizing "walking school buses" for students who wished to walk to school, publishing obesity prevention messages in a local newspaper, and sponsoring Muevete (Move) aerobics classes for Latina mothers. In addition, this case describes efforts at changing local and state policies to promote healthy eating, a critical element of social-justice-focused health promotion initiatives.

Several highly culturally contextualized programs unique to Humboldt Park have resulted. CO-OP takes a four-pronged approach to excessive weight: (1) mobilize community leaders and organizations; (2) support development of collaborations that embrace a variety of intervention projects; (3) promote healthy foods and physical exercise; and (4) link clinical practice to community programs. A steering committee is the central mechanism for implementing these strategies.

The CO-OP HP was established in 2004, based at the Puerto Rican Cultural Center Juan Antonio Corretjer. The high rates of community obesity have been addressed through five nutrition and physical activity interventions: (1) Buen Provecho (a program to help local Latino restaurants provide healthier menu options); (2) Conueco Farmers' Market on Paseo Boricua; (3) ProduceMobile (a monthly distribution of fresh fruits and vegetables in the community); (4) Muevete (an aerobics program for all ages and levels of fitness); (5) fresh produce distribution (monthly distribution of culturally preferred fresh produce).

The above projects are in various stages of development and evaluation. However, what becomes very evident is that local community characteristics (such as the Puerto Rican community in the case of Humboldt Park) bring a strong cultural dimension to projects. These projects emphasize the institutions that residents come into contact with on a regular basis, and activities that incorporate cultural traditions related to food, music, and dance. These activities would be manifested in other ways in some of Chicago's other neighborhoods of color. The tailoring of interventions to local circumstances is a hallmark of health promotion.

Coalitions such as the CO-OP HP can have significant impact on overweight and obesity when they decentralize activities to the community or neighborhood level and are sufficiently flexible to incorporate unique cultural traditions in their strategies. In other words, these activities are not one-size-fits-all. This puts tremendous pressure on the coordinating bodies to provide technical supports and interpret a wide variety of activities, their significance, and evaluation findings to their funding sources.

Case Example: Baltimore City Food Policy Task Force

The case of the Baltimore City Food Policy Task Force highlights a different form of coalition, this one seeking changes in the community by stressing the role and importance of stakeholders—here predominantly at the governmental and major organizational levels—in addressing community concerns about childhood overweight and obesity. This case does not rely heavily upon resident participation but does draw on community institutions such as grocery stores.

In 2006 the city of Baltimore discovered that residents had deep concerns about the lack of access to healthy foods that were also affordable (Hodgson, 2009). In 2007 the Johns Hopkins University School of Public Health released the findings of a study that confirmed resident concerns; it found that more than two-thirds of all adults and 40 percent of all high school students were either overweight or obese. The study results set the stage for the establishment of a city initiative focused on obesity and the ecological forces that increase weight and limit access to healthy foods and physical exercise.

The mayor established a task force composed of 15 people from city government, a university, grocery stores, and food retail associations at the city and state levels. The mission of the task force was to increase access to healthy foods (Hodgson, 2009, p. 6): "The Baltimore City Food Policy Task Force brings together stakeholders in Baltimore's food production, distribution, and consumption system to identify means to create demand for healthy food through awareness and education and to ensure opportunities for all Baltimoreans to access affordable healthy food options in order to achieve and sustain better health outcomes and a higher quality of life."

This mission statement led to the development of seven goals (Hodgson, 2009, p. 7):

1. Increase food security and accessibility for all Baltimoreans; 2. Create policies and regulations that foster and do not impede access to healthy and affordable food; 3. Create opportunities for the sale, purchase, and distribution of healthy and affordable foods; 4. Develop programs that promote the sale and consumption of healthy foods; 5. Communicate a strategic and clear message about the benefits of and opportunities for eating healthy foods; 6. Ensure that food services provided by governmental programs offer and promote healthy food choices; and 7. Reduce poor public health outcomes associated with low consumption of healthy food such as childhood obesity, heart disease, etc.

The task force recommended the following 10 strategies to promote healthy eating as a means of reducing childhood obesity:

1. Promote and Expand Farmers' Markets;
2. Promote and Expand Community Supported Agriculture;
3. Support Continued Research on Food Deserts and Collaboration with Policymakers;
4. Support a Central Kitchen Model for the Baltimore City Public School System;
5. Support Community Gardens and Urban Agriculture;
6. Expand Supermarket Home Delivery Program;
7. Improve the Food Environment around Schools and Recreation Centers;

8. Support Street Vending of Healthy Foods;
9. Create Healthy Food Zoning Requirements or Incentives; and
10. Develop a targeted marketing campaign to encourage Healthy Eating among all Baltimoreans.

The broadening of a food task force to include a focus on the built environment and physical exercise is a rare occurrence (Baltimore City Food Policy Task Force, 2009, p. 8):

> Most city governments working on food system issues have not included organizations working on increasing physical activity into their strategic framework. We think it's because often the task of getting support from food system stakeholders is so overwhelming that the thought of including another content area would mean a slowing down of progress. We recognize there needs to be an overt link in order for both programs to be effective.

Baltimore accomplished this by including the Department of Parks and Recreation as a member of the task force. The importance of the political power wielded by the mayor's office and the various city agencies that participated on the task force must be acknowledged.

Coalitions and task forces have the potential to bring together constituencies that normally may not work together. Further, they have the potential to attract increased publicity for the problem of overweight and obesity and thereby to generate external resources that can be used to create community-focused interventions. The two cases described in this chapter provide a glimpse into the richness of such types of intervention. As social workers, particularly those who are educated in community practice, we understand the value, rewards, and challenges of working in communities.

Communities represent the most promising arena in which to combat excessive weight and its consequences. Community partnerships, however, must extend beyond conventional definitions. Partnering with local food establishments, for example, can increase healthy food consumption if financial and institutional supports are built into community food initiatives (Arrom, 2006a). Active engagement of grocery store owners, based upon assessment of perceived barriers and motivators, is essential to achieve goals of increased access to healthy foods and decreased stocking of unhealthy foods (Song et al., 2010).

Evaluation Rewards and Challenges

Frank and Di Ruggiero (2003) stress the importance of careful evaluation of community-based health promotion interventions. Cheadle and colleagues (2010, p. 2130), however, note that community-level obesity prevention initiatives that stress environmental approaches are fraught with a lack of empirical evidence of their success: "The lack of existing evidence about the effectiveness of environmental interventions makes it critical to carefully evaluate the growing number of community initiatives targeting environmental change." This criticism is certainly debated. However, we must understand the relatively short history these types of interventions have enjoyed. Consequently, we must hope that progress in this arena will bring advances in research and evaluation (Cheadle et al., 2010).

Multifaceted health promotion initiatives, particularly those sponsored by community coalitions, facilitate a much-needed comprehensive approach to the problem of overweight and obesity, including the ability to measure environmental-focused interventions. Though such efforts have the potential to create innovations and empower communities, their impact can also be difficult to measure (Whitacre, Burns, Liverman, and Parker, 2009).

The story of the Community Organizing for Obesity Prevention in Humboldt Park (CO-OP HP) illustrates how gathering locally generated data on overweight and obesity can be facilitated through coalitions with active and meaningful resident involvement. Obtaining the "buy-in" from the community is essential if appropriate baseline data are to be obtained and used to measure the effectiveness of an intervention. Another example is the Houston Can Do childhood obesity prevention initiative, which also highlights both the role and the importance of qualitative data gathered at the community level and the importance of community-based coalitions in the design and implementation of a community-based program (Correa et al., 2010).

Community-based initiatives that utilize social justice perspectives as a guiding principle must allow community groups to join evaluators who stress participatory evaluation, and must include community participation as a part of the evaluation effort (Fetterman and Wandersman, 2004; Flores, 2008; Preskill and Catambas, 2006; Suarez-Balcazar and Harper, 2004). Empowerment evaluation specifically builds in community decision making and participation as a means of helping to ensure that answers to the evaluation questions meet the needs of community residents. This stress on participatory democracy ties in with social-justice-influenced overweight and obesity interventions. Rarely will evaluation findings be sufficient to achieve social change. Social change requires social action by communities with the assistance of professionals and community-based organizations (Whitacre et al., 2009).

Granner and Sharpe (2004) note that though community coalitions and partnerships are frequently recommended to address health issues such as those related to overweight and obesity, the field has not paid sufficient attention to the development of valid and reliable measurement tools. Ammerman and colleagues (2007) strongly recommend development of measurements at a community level rather than focusing on individuals, since it is not possible to track change at the individual level. Ansari and Weiss (2005) note the numerous challenges that are encountered in evaluating these types of partnerships, and issue a call for multi-method approaches that are grounded in the community where the coalitions operate.

Coalitions bring a host of rewards and challenges to any evaluation effort (Butterfoss and Francisco, 2004; Israel et al., 2006). The challenges, unfortunately, are unavoidable, but there is much that we can do to minimize the difficulties. Trust, for example, has been identified as a key element in the success of working relationships between community residents and institutions, particularly academic institutions (White-Cooper, Dawkins, and Anderson, 2009). Any social worker who has worked in marginalized urban communities would understand the level of distrust that residents may have toward large institutions.

Trust, along with leadership and efficiency, has been identified as a critical factor in coalition synergy (Jones and Barry, 2011). Becker, Longjohn, and Christoffel (2008, p. 205), who have experience in building community coalitions in Chicago, offer advice on engendering trust: "Expect all partners to act true to their identities. Academic institutions, community-based organizations, and corporate entities all have cultures that are unique unto themselves. If these unique identities are acknowledged and respected, communication and collaboration across sectors are possible. Appropriate processes for such communication and collaboration are essential."

A study of community partnerships sponsored by the Centers for Disease Control identified nine factors that are common to successful coalitions: (1) trust relationships, (2) equitable processes, (3) diverse membership, (4) all parties benefiting, (5) balance between partnership process, activities, and outcomes, (6) community involvement, (7) supportive organizational policies, (8) leadership at all levels, and (9) competent and skilled staff (Huberty et al., 2010; Seifer, 2006).

Butterfoss (2006), in turn, identified eight key process evaluation indicators that must be measured in any effort to understand the role and success of community coalitions: (1) diversity of membership, (2) recruitment of new members and retention of original membership, (3) roles in the coalition and activity participation, (4) the number of events sponsored, (5) amount of time spent in and outside of coalition activities and events, (6) benefits and challenges encountered in participating, (7) degree of satisfaction gained through participation, and (8) the balance of power and leadership.

Brownell (2007, p. 124) brings up another often overlooked aspect of the value of evaluation in community-led overweight and obesity initiatives: "Encouraging consumers to express their voice, to organize, to be creative, to evaluate the impact of local programs, and to share their results with others may be an effective means of facilitating broad changes." Sharing strategies and results becomes a vehicle through which extra-community networking and change efforts can occur.

Whitacre and colleagues (2009) identified six key challenges that evaluators face in measuring the effectiveness of community-based initiatives targeting overweight and obesity: (1) the need for consensus on measurements; (2) obtaining long-term commitment from funders to measure long-term outcomes; (3) development of new research models that are conducive to community-based interventions; (4) reducing the onus of evaluation on over-studied population groups; (5) creating new approaches to reduce excessive burden associated with complex multifactorial evaluation models; and (6) creating opportunities for publication of evaluation findings.

Finally, Cheadle and colleagues (2010, p. 2132) raise particular concerns about population-level measures:

Population-level measures are imperfect in capturing the impact of environmental [ecological] interventions on obesity. Population-level surveys are expensive to conduct, and it is difficult to obtain response rates that are representative of the entire population of a community. More importantly, it is difficult for a single intervention or even a combination of interventions to achieve a measurable population-level impact because most of these interventions are small relative to the array of factors that shape physical activity and dietary behaviors.

These and other challenges, however, take on even greater significance when community-based interventions are premised on social justice principles and actively embrace communities as leading these efforts. Thus, each of these challenges brings the added dimension of participatory democracy to deliberations.

Community-based initiatives can span a wide continuum. At one end, community is the setting for an intervention, but no substantial effort is made to involve residents. At the opposite end, community-led initiatives engage residents in critical decision-making roles or even have residents leading the effort.

Community-based approaches toward overweight and obesity can easily include community gardens and youth-led initiatives, as described earlier. However, community-based initiatives can also be structured so that communities are the context, target, and vehicle for addressing overweight and obesity. The special role that community coalitions can play has the potential to bring together a variety of community institutions in pursuit of a common goal.

The problem of overweight and obesity in urban low-income communities of color is of a magnitude that necessitates comprehensive strategies. Coalitions represent an ideal vehicle by which to include all of the significant community sectors and sustain efforts over an extended period of time. Effective coalitions, however, are labor-intensive and must be approached with careful attention to the myriad forces that may operate to undermine their potential.

13

Implications for Social Work Practice and Research

There is never an appropriate justification for treating a group of individuals poorly. Stigmatization hurts on an individual level and on a societal level. Weight bias perpetuates institutionalized problems that make it difficult to address the health disparities relevant to solving the crisis.

(POMERANZ, 2008, P. S100)

This final chapter highlights the interconnectedness of values, theory, and field examples, the implications for social work practice, and the appropriateness of employing a social justice lens. Pomeranz's (2008) poignant charge to society to pass obesity- and weight-bias laws challenges the social work profession to be a part of this movement.

The social work profession occupies a unique position from which to address the problem of overweight and obesity—from individual, family, group, organizational, community, and policy perspectives. Social justice themes serve as a foundation of social work practice in marginalized urban communities of color. The case studies and examples that have been featured here, along with the research and scholarly literature discussed, will serve as the basis for noting seven key, cross-cutting themes that have direct implications for social work.

Community Participation

The concept of empowerment has a long history in social work, whether it refers to individuals, groups, or communities. Empowerment, however, can be achieved only through the active and substantive participation of those whom we wish to assist. Community participation is about members of marginalized groups' achieving empowerment in their lives and determining how best to address the issue of obesity and excessive weight. Interventions should be planned not *for* communities, but rather *with* them.

Communities have distinct geographical dimensions as well as dimensions of ethnicity, race, and socioeconomic class. Though communities can be defined in a number of other ways as well, most practitioners and researchers tend to embrace geography and population characteristics as key elements in any definition of what constitutes community.

The detailed case examples presented reflect various degrees of community participation, and illustrate how various community subgroups can dictate how excessive weight can best be addressed within their respective communities. In all these instances, communities had a role in shaping the interventions that would affect them. All of the communities participated, to varying degrees. The central premise of this book has been that communities should be active participants, to the maximum degree possible.

Assets of Marginalized Communities

Every marginalized urban community has assets, regardless of the extent of social and health problems caused by overweight and obesity. Social workers are well versed in strengths and assets paradigms. However, other helping professions are only now warming up to the central premise that all communities have indigenous resources that can be marshaled in service to the community.

The case examples serve as testaments to the role and importance of community assets in the lives of residents, and clearly illustrate why any community-focused intervention on overweight and obesity must identify and build upon these assets if it is to be successful. How a community's assets are manifested depends very much upon local circumstances. Thus, identification, assessment, and mobilization of the available resources must be a part of any community initiative to address excess weight.

Program Evaluation

It seems impossible to conduct a community evaluation effort on overweight or obesity without encountering numerous methodological and political challenges along the way. However, it would be a stretch of the imagination to think that evaluation of community obesity interventions could be flawless in execution. Program evaluations of the types of intervention discussed in the case examples (youth interventions, community gardens, and community-led programs) all encountered challenges, but these were met through community partnerships with various significant entities. This process, particularly when it utilizes qualitative data, is labor-intensive, but well worth the time and effort. Participatory evaluation has a bright future in the field of overweight and obesity.

Social Justice and Obesity

The influence of a social justice perspective permeates the entire process of planning, implementing, and evaluating community-based excessive-weight interventions. The forces that have facilitated or even promoted excessive weight gain among select population groups are quite formidable. Social work as a profession does not have the financial resources and the political support that these industries enjoy. This comment is not intended to discourage those of us who wish to make a significant contribution in this field. It is meant, however, to suggest that we should view the challenges as a marathon rather than a hundred-meter dash. It has taken decades for our nation and communities to reach this crisis stage. It would be foolish for us to think it can be "solved" in a short period of time!

Schools as Part of the Community

Any intervention with comprehensive goals cannot afford to treat school systems as separate from the community. Schools are an integral part of the community; efforts to address excessive weight in the one cannot ignore the other. The Philadelphia public school system's decision to ban unhealthy foods and drinks in the schools and to encourage neighborhood stores to stock healthy snacks is a fine example of this. Enforcement of physical education requirements, too, should be a part of any comprehensive strategy for addressing overweight and obesity among children and youth.

Social workers should not assume that practice in schools can be carried out only by school social workers and community interventions can be carried out by community social workers. Collaboration should not just be cross-disciplinary; it should also be intra-disciplinary, with social workers collaborating across domains. School settings, in addition, lend themselves to family-centered interventions, and as a result, are not intended to be exclusively focused on students.

The Role of Social Work

The case illustrations highlight the secondary role of social work in addressing excessive weight in marginalized urban communities. This kind of participation does not supplant one-on-one work in the field, and that mode of service delivery is not to be minimized. Yet social work is not actively involved in coalitions and other organized bodies, research, and scholarship on obesity. The profession can easily play an important role at all levels of intervention and prevention, including being a part of coalitions, task forces, and social justice campaigns.

This theme is of particular concern to me because this problem is front and center to our mission. Numerous points of entry are available to the profession, including being a part of social-justice-inspired campaigns that focus especially on various corporate sectors.

Cultural Competence

This cross-cutting theme is certainly not surprising. All of the interventions discussed here related to research, theory, and case illustrations and stress the importance of contextualization if they are to be successful. Culture, in this instance, is not restricted to race and ethnicity but encompasses age, urban location, gender, and socioeconomic class, as well as other factors.

The quest for cultural competence is not restricted to obesity-related interventions. Nevertheless, it is especially significant on this topic. Unlike drugs and many other social problems, food has a strong cultural component and is thereby much more imbued with cultural beliefs, values, and traditions. This both destigmatizes the discussion of food and presents the challenge of changing nutritional behavior patterns. The importance of culture, fortunately, has long been recognized in social work, making it easier for us to modify assessment and intervention strategies to accommodate cultural uniqueness.

These seven cross-cutting themes provide valuable insights for those in social work and other helping professions as they strive to gain an in-depth understanding of the rewards and challenges associated with having communities play an instrumental role in efforts to reduce and prevent excessive weight in urban communities of color. I sincerely hope that none of the themes identified here came as any great surprise to the reader. It is important that these themes be reinforced in the process of developing effective interventions and research in this field.

Epilogue

Cities are vibrant entities, the centers for ideas and production. Cities are more than mere economic centers, they are places where people share experiences; cities are centers of innovation.
(LEVINE, 2012, P. IV)

It is appropriate to begin this epilogue with a quote that casts cities in a positive light, since all too often statements about urban areas tend to focus on their ills. The epilogue offers me a final opportunity to highlight key themes and issues that I believe will shape the debate and corresponding strategies to address overweight and obesity from this decade into the next.

Is Obesity a Crisis, Problem, Concern, or Epidemic?

The way we define the social phenomenon of obesity is obviously important; it has serious social, economic, and political ramifications. In other words, this is much more serious than an academic exercise. I am inclined to label it an epidemic because of the magnitude of the problem and the prospect that it will only get worse if we continue to fail to provide funding initiatives with these population groups as high priority.

I do welcome more active and serious debate about the labeling process because such actions help us better understand the nature of this problem and draw parallels with other major social problems (such as HIV/AIDS). However, this discussion must be expanded beyond academics and researchers to include communities and what they think the problem should be called. Labeling it an epidemic may not sit well when there are other "more pressing" epidemics in their lives, such as drugs, violence, and unemployment.

Obesity as an Issue of National Defense

We rarely think of national defense in terms other than threats from foreign powers or terrorists. Yet Levenstein (1993) titles one of the chapters in his book *Paradox of Plenty* "Oh, What a Healthy War: Nutrition for National Defense." The chapter chronicles World War II efforts at food conservation, yet the title provokes an interesting discussion.

What would we call national defense or security when a significant part of our population is slowly killing itself—and being helped to do so by established institutions? I call it a threat to national security. The ability of a nation's population to succeed and achieve a high level of well-being is critical to a nation's survival, and by that definition the crisis of overweight and obesity is clearly a threat.

America's position in the global economy is threatened when a significant portion of its population, because of health conditions, cannot help the nation compete. I would prefer to look at obesity from a non-economic standpoint. However, if money makes the world go around, we will have to argue about how the money spent on treating obesity can be better spent fostering economic projects that help this nation compete in the twenty-first century.

As a social worker I would rather see this nation address excessive weight from a rights perspective. Declaring a national war on obesity has too many similarities to a national war on crime, drugs, and poverty, and we all know that those "wars" have been lost. I also feel that establishing White House task forces on obesity and declaring a month devoted to childhood obesity do not convey the sense of urgency that is needed.

Obesity as Genocide?

The reader may think that this statement is over the top. However, what could we call a situation in which groups of individuals have been targeted for slow extinction? That, I am afraid, is what is happening in inner cities across this country. No group of color, gender, or age has escaped the onslaught. Although the issue of excessive weight casts a cloud over the entire country, there is no denying that certain groups have a higher likelihood than others of being affected. With minor exceptions, government at all levels has stood by and allowed this situation to develop, citing personal choice, profits, and jobs as justifications for inaction.

The profound social, economic, political, and health consequences of obesity, and the techniques by which the corporate sector has purposefully targeted low-income people of color, support classifying the issue of obesity as genocide. The close relationship that the food industry has cultivated with these communities as consumers and employees stands as testimony to that industry's influence, and its systematic efforts at lobbying our elected officials further make this view even less sensational.

Labeling the problem of excessive weight in low-income urban communities of color as "genocide" will undoubtedly generate a great deal of discussion and debate, which in my opinion is one of the benefits of using such a label. It is not a label I have ever used before in any of my writings even though I have devoted my professional life to working with urban communities of color. Nevertheless, we are at a critical point, and I do not want to see another generation saddled with a host of consequences because we were afraid of calling this a form of genocide.

Professional Opportunities in Fighting Obesity

Some claim that the obesity panic is largely being fueled by lobbying groups with vested interests in bringing greater attention to this problem because of the funding that it attracts. Academics, unfortunately, have been labeled as one of those groups. Social work, like other helping professions, is not immune to the temptation of funding research and scholarship agendas. Consequently, we must be careful of signing on to help eradicate excessive weight without serious debate about our participation in this "industry."

I am particularly concerned about what I perceive to be a disturbing trend in schools of social work that views the acquisition of external funding by a faculty member as a key factor, if not the only factor, that determines whether that scholar is productive and deserving of tenure and promotion. An emphasis on research that can generate external funding, with its corresponding overhead, can prove quite troubling when the social work *Code of Ethics* mandates that practitioners address oppression and seek social justice goals.

Those who examine issues such as obesity from a social justice perspective are bound to encounter problems in getting funding from government entities and major foundations. Thus, academics with secured positions are the only ones left to pursue this line of inquiry. Merit increases for that small group will be limited because of the lack of external funding. Obviously, the decision to pursue obesity-related funding that is apolitical will be an individual decision. However, I do not believe that the support of scholarship from a social justice perspective will ever approach that from a non–social justice perspective, and thus the potential contributions that social work and other helping professions can make to obesity-related knowledge will be limited.

Community First and Foremost

The "people first" movement, which sought to ensure that people with various disabilities were considered people first, serves as an excellent guide for our efforts at addressing overweight and obesity. One of the strengths of social work as a profession is its historical emphasis on viewing community as context and as a vehicle for achieving significant change. In the case of excessive weight and marginalized communities, this emphasis also serves as a vehicle for empowering the beneficiaries of interventions to shape the goals and methods of those interventions.

There is little doubt that any significant progress in addressing excessive weight among marginalized urban groups will be accomplished at the community level, by focusing on individuals. Communities must play a vital decision-making role in designing and implementing initiatives. We must ensure that this criterion is met as we venture into coalitions and partnerships with professions that do not have a history of community practice. Such a position does not mean that we have found truth and now will help others find it. It does mean that it is not possible to find truth without a meaningful focus on communities.

The Importance of Prevention

The problem of excessive weight has most commonly been addressed from a treatment perspective. However, waiting for overweight and obesity to manifest itself in hospitals and community health centers is financially unwise and has regrettable and preventable impacts on daily living and well-being. Consequently, social workers, in collaboration with other professions and communities, must advocate for prevention.

The measurement of prevention effectiveness is not easy, although significant progress has been made. The complexity of weight gain is compounded by focusing on communities as an entity and how specific subgroups view excessive weight. Community-based research is complex and time-consuming because of the importance of relationships in establishing the requisite foundation for prevention projects.

Beyond the Box: Coalitions and Non-traditional Settings

Community coalitions involving community residents and institutions are undeniably crucial to the effort. It is important to emphasize, however, that potential coalitions should not be restricted to formal social service organizations. We must expand our vision to include non-traditional settings (Delgado, 1999).

Non-traditional settings are places in a community where residents congregate for business or social reasons. They may also be places where residents receive some form of social services. Non-traditional settings can be houses of worship, grocery stores, restaurants, beauty parlors, and bakeries. These establishments must also be considered as potential partners in any coalition to combat excessive weight. Though they will rarely, if ever, appear in a resource directory of local service organizations, they wield a great deal of influence in the daily life of communities. Prominent members of these organizations, including local business owners, can be an effective part of community coalitions and campaigns to achieve healthy eating habits and exercise. Community resources, both formal and informal, expand a community's assets to a broader perspective.

The Interplay of Food, Exercise, and Genetics

Finally, to what extent are overweight and obesity the result of overeating, lack of physical exercise, and/or a genetic predisposition toward excessive weight? Billions of dollars are at stake, depending on how this question is answered and who is being asked to answer it. Multiple industries (diet, medical, and research in particular) have a vested interest in shaping the response to the question.

It is clear that no one dimension is totally responsible for overweight and obesity. Genetics does play a role, but that is beyond the control of interventions at this point in time. It is important, however, not to equate genetics with destiny. We certainly can control food access and physical exercise for those who have a genetic predisposition toward excessive weight.

Concentrating on these two areas will go a long way toward helping to reduce overweight and obesity in this country in general, and in urban communities of color in particular. Yet both of these manageable factors are influenced by powerful industry lobbying groups that have shown significant and ongoing resistance to any attempt to interfere with their billion-dollar profits. The elimination of parks and recreation programs, for example, has often been advocated for as a means of cutting governmental costs, and this is shortsighted.

Despite the numerous challenges facing the field of excessive-weight prevention, we cannot take a "business as usual" approach to addressing the issue in urban marginalized communities if we hope to save a generation from the deleterious consequences associated with this condition.

The field of health promotion, particularly as it relates to overweight and obesity, is ever expanding, bringing with that growth a host of new rewards and new challenges. The introduction of social work as a participating profession in the field represents but the latest chapter in its evolution. I would like to think that our involvement will lead not only to more relevance for marginalized population groups but also to more effectiveness in reducing excessive weight and mitigating its consequences for countless people across this nation.

References

Abraham, A., Sommerhalder, K., and Abel, T. (2010). Landscape and well-being: A scoping study on the health-promoting impact of outdoor environments. *International Journal of Public Health*, 55, no. 1: 59–69.

Addy, C. L., Wilson, D. K., Kirtland, K. A., Ainsworth, B. E., Sharp, P., and Kimsey, D. (2004). Associations of perceived social and physical environmental supports with physical activity and walking behavior. *American Journal of Public Health*, 94, no. 3: 440–443.

Adler, N. E., and Stewart, J. (2009). Reducing obesity: Motivating action while not blaming the victim. *Milbank Quarterly*, 87, no. 1: 49–70.

Agyeman, J. (2005). *Sustainable communities and the challenge of environmental justice.* New York: New York University Press.

Aicken, C., Arai, L., and Roberts, H. (2008). *Schemes to promote healthy weight among obese and overweight children in England. Report.* London: EPPI-Centre, Social Science Research Unit, Institute of Education, University of London.

Aitken, S. C. (2001). *Geographies of young people: The morally contested spaces of identity.* New York: Routledge.

Akresh, I. R. (2008). Overweight and obese foreign-born and U.S.-born Hispanics. *Biodemography and Social Biology*, 54, no. 2: 183–199.

Alaimo, K., Packnett, E., Miles, R. A., and Kruger, D. J. (2008). Fruit and vegetable intake among urban community gardeners. *Journal of Nutrition Education and Behavior*, 40, no. 2: 94–101.

Ali, S. (2011, March 2). Obesity crisis: How the food industry profits while society pays. *DiversityInc.* http://diversityinc.com/article/7530/Obesity-Crisis-How-the-Food-Industry-Profits-While- . . . Accessed 4/11/11.

Alkon, A. (2008). Paradise or pavement: The social constructions of the environment in two urban farmers' markets and their implications for environmental justice and sustainability. *Local Environment: The International Journal of Justice and Sustainability*, 13, no. 3: 271–289.

Alkon, A. H., and Norgaard, K. M. (2009). Breaking the food chains: An investigation of food justice activism. *Sociological Inquiry*, 79, no. 3: 289–305.

Allday, E. (2010, July 8). Another way to lose weight—impose a 20% tax on soda. *San Francisco Chronicle*, p. A10.

Allen, J. (2002). The role of mentoring in health promotion. *American Journal of Health Promotion*, 17, no. 1: 1–7.

Allen, O. J., Alaimo, K., Doris, E., and Perry, E. (2008). Growing vegetables and values: Benefits of neighborhood-based community gardens for youth development and nutrition. *Journal of Hunger and Environmental Nutrition*, 3, no. 4: 418–439.

Allen, P. (2008). Mining for justice in the food system: Perceptions, practices, and possibilities. *Agriculture and Human Values*, 25, no. 2: 157–161.

Allen, P., Dusen, D. V., Lundy, J., and Gliessman, S. (1991). Integrating social, environmental, and economic issues in sustainable agriculture. *American Journal of Alternative Agriculture*, 6, no. 1: 34–39.

Allen, P., and Sachs, C. (2007). Women and food chains: The gendered politics of food. *International Journal of Sociology of Food and Agriculture*, 15, no. 1: 1–23.

Allison, D. B., Downey, M., Atkinson, R. L., Billington, C. J., Bray, G. A., Eckel, R. H., Finkelstein, E. A., Jensen, M. D., and Tremblay, A. (2008). Obesity as a disease: A white paper on evidence and arguments commissioned by the Council of the Obesity Society. *Obesity*, 16, no. 6: 1161–1177.

Allison, D. B., Nathan, J. S., Albu, J. B., Heymsfield, S. B., Dupral, L. T., and Pi-Sunyer, F. X. (1998). Measurement challenges and other practical concerns when studying massively obese individuals. *International Journal of Eating Disorders*, 24, no. 3: 275–284.

Alvanides, S., Townshend, T. G., and Lake, A. A. (2010). Obesogenic environments: Challenges and opportunities. In A. A. Lake, T. G. Townshend, and S. Alvanides (Eds.), *Obesogenic environments: Complexities, perceptions, and objective measures* (pp. 215–220). Oxford, UK: Blackwell Publishing.

Alvaro, C., Jackson, L. A., Kirk, S., McHugh, T. L., Huges, J., Chircop, A., and Lyons, R. F. (2010). Moving Canadian governmental policies beyond a focus on individual lifestyle: Some insights from complexity and critical theories. *Health Promotion International*, 26, no. 1: 91–99.

American Medical Association Council on Scientific Affairs. (1999). *Obesity as a major public health problem.* Report 6. American Medical Association annual meeting.

Ammerman, A.S., Samuel-Hodge, C. D., Sommers, J. K., Leung, M. M., Paxton, A. E., and Vu, M. B. (2007). Community-based approaches to obesity prevention: The role of environmental and policy change. In S. Kumanyika and R. C. Brownson (Eds.), *Handbook of obesity prevention: A resource for health professionals* (pp. 263–284). New York: Springer.

Anandacoomarasamy, A., Caterson, I., Sambrook, P., Fransen, M., and March, L. (2008). The impact of obesity on the musculoskeletal system: Obesity and musculoskeletal disease. *International Journal of Obesity*, 32, no. 2: 211–222.

Anderson, M. D. (2008). Rights-based food systems and the goals of food systems reform. *Agriculture and Human Values*, 25, no. 2: 593–608.

Anderson, M. D., and Cook, J. T. (1999). Community food security: Practice in need of theory? *Agriculture and Human Values*, 16, no. 3: 141–150.

Anderson, P. (2009, August 27). Hispanics have double the complication rate after carotid surgery. *Medscape News*.

Andreyeva, T., Puhl, R. M., and Brownell, K. D. (2008). Changes in perceived weight discrimination among Americans, 1955–1996 through 2004–2006. *Behavior and Psychology*, 16, no. 5: 1129–1134.

Ansari, W. E., and Weiss, E. S. (2005). Quality of research on community partnerships: Developing the evidence base. *Health Education Research*, 21, no. 3: 175–180.

Aranceta, J., Moreno, B., Moya, M., and Anadon, A. (2009). Prevention of overweight and obesity from a public health perspective. *Nutrition Review*, 67, suppl. 1: S83–S88.

Aranda, M. P. (2006). Older Latinos: A mental health perspective. In B. Berkman (Ed.), *Handbook of social work in health and aging* (pp. 283–292). New York: Oxford University Press.

Ariza, A. J., Chen, E. H., Binns, H. J., and Christoffel, K. K. (2004). Risk factors for overweight in five- to six-year-old Hispanic-American children: A pilot study. *Journal of Urban Health*, 81, no. 1: 150–161.

Armstrong, D. (2000). A survey of community gardens in upstate New York: Implications for health promotion and community development. *Health and Place*, 6, no. 4: 319–327.

Armstrong, D. (2011, July 8). Obesity rates rise at least 90% in 17 states since 1995, study says. *Boston Globe*, p. A11.

Arredondo, E., Castaneda, D., Elder, J. P., Slymen, D., and Dozier, D. (2009). Brand name logo recognition of fast food and healthy food among children. *Journal of Community Health*, 34, no. 1: 73–78.

Arrom, J. O. (2006a). *Promoting healthy eating in the Latino South Chicago neighborhood: An ecological approach.* Paper presented at the American Public Health Association annual meeting, Boston, MA.

Arrom, J. O. (2006b). *Design and participatory evaluation of gardening intervention to prevent childhood obesity: Bush Community Gardens of Hope.* Paper presented at the American Public Health Association annual meeting, Boston, MA.

Ash, M., Boyce, J. K., Chang, G., and Scharber, H. (2010). *Is environmental justice good for white folk?* Amherst, MA: Political Economy Research Institute, University of Massachusetts.

Associated Press. (2011, May 12). Cameras to measure what students eat. *Boston Globe*, p. A2.

Ayala, G. X., Mueller, K., Lopez-Madurga, E., Campbell, N., and Elder, J. P. (2005). Restaurant and food shopping selections among Latino women in Southern California. *Journal of the American Dietetic Association*, 105, no. 1: 38–45.

Ayala, G. X., Rogers, M., Arredondo, E. M., Campbell, N. R., Baquero, B., Duerkson, S. C., and Elder, T. P. (2008). Away-from-home food intake and the risk for obesity: Examining the influence of context. *Obesity*, 16, no. 5: 1002–1008.

Azuma, A. M., Gilliland, S., Vallianatos, M., and Gottlieb, G. (2010). Food access, availability, and affordability in 3 Los Angeles communities, Project CAFE, 2004–2006. *Preventing Chronic Disease*, 7, no. 2: 1–9.

Baines, M., Dixon, E., Lewis, D., Liu, Y., MacFarland, M., Pritchett, L., Singletary, R., and Tiver, S. (2010). *Community gardens*. Danville, VA: Danville Regional Foundation.

Baker, E. L. (2004). Tending cultural landscapes and food citizenship in Toronto's community gardens. *Geographical Review*, 94, no. 3: 305–325.

Ball, K., Crawford, D., Timperio, A., and Salmon, J. (2010). Eating behaviors and the food environment. In A. A. Lake, T. G. Townshend, and S. Alvanides (Eds.), *Obesogenic environments: Complexities, perceptions, and objective measures* (pp. 149–163). Oxford, UK: Blackwell Publishing.

Baltimore City Food Policy Task Force. (2009). *Final report and recommendations*. Baltimore, MD: Author.

Barr, D. A. (2008). *Health disparities in the United States: Social class, race, ethnicity, and health*. Baltimore, MD: The Johns Hopkins University Press.

Barroso, C. S., Peters, R. J., Johnson, R. J., Kelder, S. H., and Jefferson, T. (2010). Beliefs and perceived norms concerning body image among African-American and Latino teenagers. *Journal of Health Psychology*, 15, no. 6: 858–870.

Barusch, A. S. (2009). *Foundations of social policy: Social justice in human perspective* (3rd ed.). Belmont, CA: Brooks/Cole.

Bates, L. M., Acevedo-Garcia, D., Alegria, M., and Krieger, N. (2008). Immigration and generational trends in body mass index and obesity in the United States: Results of the national Latino and Asian American survey, 2002–2003. *American Journal of Public Health*, 98, no. 1: 70–77.

Battisi, D. S., and Naylor, R. L. (2009). Historical warnings of future food insecurity with unprecedented seasonal heat. *Science*, 329, no. 5911: 240–244.

Baum, C. L. (2007). The effects of race, ethnicity, and age on obesity. *Journal of Population Economics*, 20, no. 6: 687–705.

Baum, C. L. (2011). The effects of food stamps on obesity. *Southern Economic Journal*, 77, no. 3: 623–651.

Baum, F. (2007). Cracking the nut of health equity: Top down and bottom up pressure for action on the social determinants of health. *Promotion and Health*, 14, no. 2: 90–97.

Becker, A. B., Longjohn, M., and Christoffel, K. K. (2008). Taking on childhood obesity in a big city: Consortium to Lower Obesity in Chicago Children (CLOCC). *Progress in Pediatric Cardiology*, 25, no. 2: 199–206.

Benforado, A., Hanson, J., and Yosifon, D. (2006). *Broken scales: Obesity and justice in America.* San Clara University School of Law Legal Studies Research Paper Series (Working paper No. 06–16).

Bennett, G. G., and Wolin, K. Y. (2006). Satisfied or unaware? Racial differences in perceived weight status. *International Journal of Behavioral Nutrition and Physical Activity*, 40, no. 3. doi:10.1186/1479–5868–3–40.

Berg, F. M. (2004). *Underage and overweight: America's childhood obesity crisis—what every family needs to know.* New York: Hatherleigh Books.

Bergman, R. N., Stefanovski, D., Buchanan, T. A., Summer, A. E., Reynolds, J. C., Sebring, N. G., Xiang, A. H., and Watanabe, R. M. (2011). A better index of body adiposity. *Obesity*, 19, no. 5: 1083–1089.

Berkman, B., and D'Ambruoso, S. (Eds.). (2006). *Handbook of social work in health and aging.* New York: Oxford University Press.

Bhattacharya, J., and Bundorf, M. K. (2009). The incidence of the healthcare costs of obesity. *Journal of Health Economics*, 28, no. 3: 649–658.

Biotech Business Week. (2010, March 29). Childhood obesity prevention is focus of Global Nutrition Transition Conference, p. 4057.

Bittman, M. (2010, February 14). A sin we sip instead of smoke? *New York Times*, p. WK1.

Black, J., and Macinko, J. (2007). Neighborhood and obesity. *Nutrition Review*, 66, no. 1: 2–20.

Blair, D. (2009). The child in the garden: An evaluative review of the benefits of school gardening. *Journal of Environmental Education*, 40, no. 2: 15–38.

Bleich, S. N., Wang, Y. C., and Gortmaker, S. L. (2009). Increasing consumption of sugar-sweetened beverages among U.S. adults: 1988–1994 to 1999–2004. *American Journal of Clinical Nutrition*, 89, no. 4: 372–381.

Boardman, J. D., St. Onge, J. M., Rogers, R., and Denney, J. T. (2005). Race differentials in obesity: The impact of place. *Journal of Health and Social Behavior*, 46, no. 3: 229–243.

Bodor, J. N., Rice, J. C., Farley, T. A., Swalm, C. M., and Rose, D. (2010). The association between obesity and urban food environments. *Journal of Urban Health*, 87, no. 5: 771–781.

Bodor, J. N., Ulmer, U. M., Dunaway, L. F., Farley, T. A., and Rose, D. (2010). The rationale behind small food store interventions in low-income urban neighborhoods: Insights from New Orleans. *Journal of Nutrition*, 140, no. 6: 1185–1188.

Boero, N. (2007). All the news that's fat to print: The American "obesity epidemic" and the media. *Qualitative Sociology*, 30, no. 1: 41–60.

Boocock, S. S., and Scott, K. A. (2005). *Kids in context: The sociological study of children and childhoods*. Lanham, MD: Rowman and Littlefield.

Boone, C. G., Buckley, G. L., Grove, M., and Sister, C. (2009). Parks and people: An environmental justice inquiry in Baltimore, Maryland. *Annals of the Association of American Geographers*, 99, no. 4: 767–787.

Booth, K. M., Pinkston, M. M., and Poston, W. S. C. (2005). Obesity and the built environment. *Journal of the American Dietetic Association*, 105, no. 5, suppl. 1: 110–117.

Borders, T. F., Rahrer, J. E., and Carderelli, K. M. (2006). Gender-specific: Disparities in obesity. *Journal of Community Health*, 31, no. 1: 57–68.

Born, B., and Purcell, M. (2006). Avoiding the local trap: Scale and food systems in planning research. *Journal of Planning Education and Research*, 26, no. 2: 195–207.

Borre, K., Ertle, L., and Graff, M. (2010). Working to eat: Vulnerability, food insecurity, and obesity among migrant and seasonal farmer families. *American Journal of Industrial Medicine*, 53, no. 4: 443–462.

Bowie, J. V., Juon, H.-S. Cho, J., and Rodriguez, M. S. (2007). Factors associated with overweight and obesity among Mexican Americans and Central Americans: Results from the 2001 California Health Interview Survey. *Preventing Chronic Disease: Public Health Research, Practice, and Policy*, 4, no. 1: 1–17.

Boylan, M., Smith, M., Borrego, J., Reed, D., Feng, D., Chyu, M., and Esperat, C. (2010). Acculturation and adiposity parameters in young Hispanic children. *Journal of the American Dietetic Association*, 110, no. 9, suppl. 1: A46.

Braithwaite, K. (2008). Health is a human right, right? *American Journal of Public Health*, 98, suppl. 1: S5–S7.

Bramble, J., Cornelius, L. J., and Simpson, G. (2009). Eating as a cultural expression of caring among Afro-Caribbean and African American women: Understanding the cultural dimensions of obesity. *Journal of Health Care for the Poor and Underserved*, 20, suppl. 2A: 53–68.

Branch, R., and Chester, A. (2009). Community-based participatory clinical research in obesity by adolescents: Pipeline for researchers of the future. *Clinical and Translational Science*, 2, no. 5: 350–354.

Brand, A. L. (2007). *Restructuring social and spatial justice in dialectical time*. Cambridge, MA: MIT Department of Urban Studies and Planning.

Brisbon, N., Plumb, J., Brawer, R., and Paxman, D. (2005). The asthma and obesity epidemics: The role played by the built environment—a public health perspective. *Journal of Allergy and Clinical Immunology*, 115, no. 5: 1024–1028.

Brodkin, K. (2009). *Power politics: Environmental activism in South Los Angeles*. New Brunswick, NJ: Rutgers University Press.

Brown, A. (2002). Farmers' market research, 1940–2000: An inventory and review. *American Journal of Alternative Agriculture*, 17, no. 2: 167–176.

Brown, C. (2010). Greenspace, obesity, and health: Evidence and issues. In A. A. Lake, T. G. Townshend, and S. Alvanides (Eds.), *Obesogenic environments: Complexities, perceptions, and objective measures* (pp. 133–147). Oxford, UK: Blackwell Publishing.

Brown, K. H., and Jameson, A. L. (2000). Public health implications of urban agriculture. *Journal of Public Health Policy*, 21, no. 1: 20–39.

Brown, N., Griffis, R., Hamilton, K., Irish, S., and Kanouse, S. (2007). What makes justice spatial? What makes spaces just?: Three interviews on the concept of spatial justice. *Critical Planning: UCLA Journal of Urban Planning*, Summer: 7–28.

Brown, P. (1992). Popular epidemiology and toxic waste contamination: Lay and professional ways of knowing. *Journal of Health and Social Behavior*, 33, no. 4: 267–281.

Brown, P. L. (2011, October 10). When the uprooted put down roots: For income and a taste of home, refugees turn to farming. *New York Times*, p. A12.

Brownell, K. D. (2007). Consumer perspectives and consumer action. In S. Kumanyika and R. C. Brownson (Eds.), *Handbook of obesity prevention: A resource for health professionals* (pp. 115–127). New York: Springer.

Brownell, K. D. (2010). Government intervention and the nation's diet: The slippery slope of inaction. *American Journal of Bioethics*, 10, no. 3: 1–2.

Brownell, K. D., and Horgen, K. B. (2006). *Food fight: The inside story of the food industry, America's obesity crisis, and what we can do about it.* Chicago: Contemporary Books.

Brownell, K. D., Kersh, R., Ludwig, D. S., Post, R. C., Puhl, R. M., Schwartz, M. B., and Willett, W. C. (2010). Personal responsibility and obesity: A constructive approach to a controversial issue. *Health Affairs*, 29, no. 3: 379–387.

Brownson, R. C., and Kumanyika, S. (2007). Obesity prevention: Charting a course to a healthier future. In S. Kumanyika and R. C. Brownson (Eds.), *Handbook of obesity prevention: A resource for health professionals* (pp. 515–528). New York: Springer.

Brulle, R. J., and Pellow, D. N. (2006). Environmental justice: Human health and environmental inequalities. *Annual Review of Public Health*, 27, no. 1: 103–123.

Buchanan, D. R., Miller, F. G., and Wallerstein, N. (2007). Balancing rigorous research with community participation in community intervention studies. *Progress in Community Health Partnerships: Research, Evaluation, and Action*, 1, no. 2: 153–160.

Budrys, G. (2003). *Unequal health: How inequality contributes to health or illness.* Lanham, MD: Rowman and Littlefield.

Buhin, L., and Vera, E. M. (2009). Preventing racism and promoting social justice: Person-centered and environment-centered interventions. *Journal of Primary Prevention*, 30, no. 1: 43–59.

Bullard, R. D. (Ed.). (2005a). *The quest for environmental justice: Human rights and the politics of pollution.* San Francisco: Sierra Club Books.

Bullard, R. D. (2005b). Environmental justice in the twenty-first century. In R. D. Bullard (Ed.), *The quest for environmental justice: Human rights and the politics of pollution* (pp. 19–42). San Francisco: Sierra Club Books.

Bullard, R. D. (2005c). Introduction. In R. D. Bullard (Ed.), *The quest for environmental justice: Human rights and the politics of pollution* (pp. 1–15). San Francisco: Sierra Club Books.

Burkhauser, R. V., and Cawley, J. (2008). Beyond BMI: The value of more accurate measures of fatness and obesity in social science research. *Journal of Health Economics*, 27, no. 2: 519–529.

Burnett, D. (2006–2007). Fast-food lawsuits and the cheeseburger bill: Critiquing Congress's response to the obesity epidemic. *Virginia Journal of Social Policy and Law*, 14:357–417.

Burns, D., Costello, J., Haggart, M., Kerr, J., Longshaw, K., and Thornton, R. (2009). The public health challenges of obesity: Is it the new smoking? *Journal of Community Nursing*, 23, no. 11: 4–9.

Burris, S., and Anderson, E. D. (2010). A framework convention on global health: Social justice lite, or light on social justice? *Journal of Law, Medicine, and Ethics*, 38, no. 3: 580–593.

Bush, C. L., Pittman, S., McKay, S., Ortiz, T., Wong, W. W., and Klish, W. (2007). Park-based obesity intervention program for inner-city children. *Journal of Pediatrics*, 151, no. 5: 513–517.

Bustillos, B., Sharkey, J. R., Anding, J., and McIntosh, A. (2009). Availability of more healthful food alternatives in traditional, convenience, and nontraditional types of food stores in two rural Texas counties. *Journal of the American Dietary Association*, 109, no. 5: 883–889.

Butterfoss, F. D. (2006). Process evaluation for community participation. *Annual Review of Public Health*, 27:323–340.

Butterfoss, F. D., and Francisco, V. T. (2004). Evaluating community partnerships and coalitions with practitioners in mind. *Health Promotion Practice*, 6, no. 2: 108–114.

Byers, T., and Sedjo, R. L. (2007). Public health response to the obesity epidemic: Too soon or too late? *Journal of Nutrition*, 137, no. 2: 488–492.

Byrne, J., Wolch, J., and Zhang, J. (2009). Planning for environmental justice in an urban national park. *Journal of Environmental Planning and Management*, 52, no. 3: 365–392.

Bywater, P. (2007). Tackling inequalities in health: A global challenge for social work. *British Journal of Social Work*, 39, no. 2: 353–367.

Cahill, M. (2010). *Transport, environment, and society*. Maidenhead, UK: Open University Press.

Cahill, S. M., and Suarez-Balcazar, Y. (2009). Promoting children's nutrition and fitness in the urban context. *American Journal of Occupational Therapy*, 63, no. 1: 113–116.

California Department of Education. (2011). *Physical fitness testing.* Sacramento: Author.

California Health Policy Forum. (2009). *Tackling obesity by building healthy communities: Changing policies through innovative collaborations.* Sacramento: Author.

CalorieLab.com. (2010). Mississippi is the fattest state in the nation for the 5th straight year and Colorado the leanest. http://calorielab.com/news/2010/06/28/fattest-states-2010/. Accessed 4/1/11.

Calzada, P. J., and Anderson-Worts, P. (2009). The obesity epidemic: Are minority individuals equally affected? *Primary Care: Clinics in Office Practice,* 35, no. 2: 307–317.

Cammarota, J. (2011). From hopelessness to hope: Social justice pedagogy in urban education and youth development. *Urban Education,* 46, no. 4: 828–844.

Campbell, M. K., Hudson, M. A., Resnicow, K., Blakeney, N., Paxton, A., and Resnicow, K. (2007). Church-based health promotion interventions: Evidence and lessons learned. *Annual Review of Public Health,* 28:213–234.

Campos, P. (2004). *The obesity myth: Why America's obsession with weight is hazardous to your health.* New York: Penguin Group.

Campos, P., Saguy, A., Ernsberger, P., Oliver, E., and Gaesser, G. (2006). The epidemiology of overweight and obesity: Public health crisis or moral panic? *International Journal of Epidemiology,* 35, no. 1: 55–60.

Canay, D., and Buchan, I. (2007). Challenges in obesity epidemiology. *Obesity Reviews,* 8, suppl. 1: 1–11.

The Cancer Project. (2008). *Cheap eats for hard times: The five most unhealthy fast food "Value Menu" items. A report from the Cancer Project.* Washington, DC: Author.

Caprio, S., Daniels, S. T., Drewnowski, A., Kaufman, F. R., Palinkas, L. A., Rosenbloom, A. L., and Schwimmer, J. B. (2008). Influence of race, ethnicity, and culture on childhood obesity: Implications for prevention and treatment. *Diabetes Care,* 31, no. 11: 2211–2221.

Caraher, M., and Covency, J. (2004). Public health nutrition and food policy. *Public Health Nutrition,* 7, no. 10: 591–598.

Cargo, M., and Mercer, S. C. (2008). The value and challenges of participatory research: Strengthening its practice. *Annual Review of Public Health,* 29:325–350.

Carr, D. M. (2007). *Effective health promotion interventions for adults of African and Caribbean descent living in urban settings: A critical exposition of the literature.* London: Queen Mary, University of London, and City University.

Carter, M. (2010). Foreword. In. D. Despommier, *The vertical farm: Feeding the world in the 21st century* (pp. ix–xiv). New York: St. Martin's Press.

Carter, S. M., Rychetnik, L., Lloyd, B., Kerridge, I. H., Baur, L., Bauman, A., and Zask, A. (2011). Evidence, ethics, and values: A framework for health promotion. *American Journal of Public Health,* 101, no. 3: 465–472.

Casagrande, S., Wang, Y., Anderson, C., and Gary, T. (2007). Have Americans increased their fruit and vegetable intake? The trends between 1988 and 2002. *American Journal of Preventive Medicine*, 32, no. 4: 257–263.

Catenacci, V. A., and Wyatt, H. R. (2007). The role of physical activity in producing and maintaining weight loss. *Nature Clinical Practice Endocrinology and Metabolism*, 3, no. 7: 518–529.

Cawley, J. (2007). The cost-effectiveness of programs to prevent or reduce obesity. *Archives of Pediatrics and Adolescent Medicine*, 161, no. 6: 611–614.

CDC (Centers for Disease Control and Prevention). (2009). *New obesity data shows Blacks have a higher rate of obesity*. Atlanta: Author.

CDC (Centers for Disease Control and Prevention). (2010a). *CDC Growth Charts: United States*. http://www.cdc.gov/growthcharts/background.htm. Accessed 7/7/10.

CDC (Centers for Disease Control and Prevention). (2010b). *REACH U.S.: Finding solutions to health disparities:* At a glance 2010. Atlanta: Author.

CDC (Centers for Disease Control and Prevention). (2010c). *Be healthy and safe in the garden.* http://www.cdc.gov/Features/GardeningTips/. Accessed 8/1/10.

CDC (Centers for Disease Control and Prevention). (2010d). *Chronic diseases and health promotion.* Atlanta: Author.

CDC (Centers for Disease Control and Prevention). (2011a). *United States obesity trends.* Atlanta: Author.

CDC (Centers for Disease Control and Prevention). (2011b). *Adult obesity.* Atlanta: Author.

CDC (Centers for Disease Control and Prevention). (2011c). *Obesity: Halting the epidemic by making health easier.* Atlanta: Author.

Chadiha, L. A., Brown, E., and Aranda, M. P. (2006). Older African American and other Black populations. In B. Berkman and S. D' Ambruoso (Eds.), *Handbook of social work in health and aging* (pp. 227–256). New York: Oxford University Press.

ChallengeDiabetes.com. (2009, March 13). Diabetes undiagnosed—high health care costs. Author.

Chambers, A. J., Sukits, A. L., McCrory, J. L., and Cham, R. (2010). The effect of obesity and gender on body segment parameters in older adults. *Clinical Biomechanics*, 25, no. 2: 131–136.

Chamorro, R., and Flores-Ortiz, Y. (2000). Acculturation and disordered eating patterns among Mexican American women. *International Journal of Eating Disorders*, 28, no. 2: 125–129.

Chaoyand, L., Ford, E. S., McGuire, L. C., and Mokdad, A. H. (2007). Increasing trends in waist circumference and abdominal obesity among U.S. adults. *Obesity*, 15, no. 1: 216–224.

Chasan-Taber, L., Schmidt, M. D., Pekow, P., Sternfeld, B., Solomon, C. G., and Markenson, G. (2008). Predictors of excessive and inadequate gestational weight gain in Hispanic women. *Epidemiology*, 16, no. 7: 1657–1666.

Chase, K. J. (2011, April 14). With demand surging, McDonald's hosts hiring event to fill 50,000 jobs. *Boston Globe*, pp. B5, B7.

Chatterjee, N., Blakely, D. E., and Barton, C. (2005). Perspectives on obesity and barriers to control from workers at a community center serving low-income Hispanic children and families. *Journal of Community Health Nursing*, 22, no. 1: 23–36.

Cheadle, A., Samuels, S. E., Rauzon, S., Yoshida, S. C., Schwartz, P. M., Boyle, M., Beery, W. L., Craypo, L., and Solomon, L. (2010). Approaches to measuring the extent and impact of environmental change in three California community-level obesity prevention initiatives. *American Journal of Public Health*, 100, no. 11: 2129–2136.

Checkoway, B. (2010). What is youth participation? *Children and Youth Services Review*, 33, no. 2: 340–345.

Chen, J.-L., Weiss, S., Heyman, M. B., and Lustig, R. (2009). Risk factors for obesity and high blood pressure in Chinese-American children: Maternal acculturation and children's food choices. *Journal of Immigrant and Minority Health*, 13, no. 2: 268–275.

Chen, S. E., Florax, R. J. G. M., and Snyder, S. D. (2009). *Obesity, fast food, and grocery stores: Evidence from geo-referenced micro data*. West Lafayette, IN: Department of Agricultural Economics, Purdue University.

Chernyak, Y., and Lowe, M. R. (2010). Motivation for dieting: Drive for thinness is different from drive for objective thinness. *Journal of Abnormal Psychology*, 119, no. 2: 276–281.

Chiolero, A., and Paccaud, F. (2009). Viewpoints: An obesity epidemic booga booga? *European Journal of Public Health*, 19, no. 6: 568–569.

Cho, J., and Juon, H.-S. (2006). Assessing overweight and obesity risk among Korean-Americans in California: Using World Health Organization Body Index Criteria for Asians. *Preventing Chronic Disease*, 3, no. 3: 1–11.

Christiansen, E. (2008). *Diabetes prevalence and prevention in African American and Hispanic populations: A review of diabetes research and prevention programs*. Reno: Center for Program Evaluation, University of Nevada College of Health and Human Services.

Christie, C., Watkins, J. A., Weerts, S., and Jackson, H. D. (2010). Community church-based intervention reduces obesity indicators in African American females. *Internet Journal of Nutrition and Wellness*, 9, no. 2: 1–17.

Christopher, G. (2008). Social justice and health outcomes in vulnerable communities. *Journal of the Medical Sciences*, 335, no. 4: 251–253.

Cintron-Moscoso, F. (2010). Cultivating youth proenvironmental development: A critical ecological approach. *Ecopsychology*, 2, no. 1: 33–40.

Clark, H. F., Bradander, D. J., and Erdil, R. M. (2006). Sources, sinks, and exposure pathways to lead in urban garden soils. *Journal of Environmental Quality*, 35, no. 6: 2066–2074.

Clifford, S. (2011, April 25). One size fits nobody: Seeking a steady 4 or a 10. *New York Times*, pp. A1, A16.

Cockerham, W. C. (2007). *Social causes of health and disease.* Cambridge, UK: Polity Press.

Cohen, S. (2003). *Folk devils and moral panic* (3rd ed.). New York: Routledge.

Colditz, G. A., and Stein, C. (2007). Costs of obesity. In S. Kumanyika and R. C. Brownson (Eds.), *Handbook of obesity prevention: A resource for health professionals* (pp. 73–83). New York: Springer.

Coleman, K. J., et al. (2010). Outcomes from a culturally tailored diabetes prevention program in Hispanic families from a low-income school: Horton Hawks Stay Healthy (HHSH). *Diabetes Educator,* 36, no. 5: 784–792.

Committee on Health Care for Underserved Women. (2010). *Challenge for overweight and obese urban women.* Washington, DC: College of Obstetricians and Gynecologists.

Connelly, J., Duaso, M., and Butler, G. (2009). A systematic review of controlled trials of interventions to prevent childhood obesity and overweight: A realistic synthesis of the evidence. *Public Health,* 121, no. 7: 510–517.

Connelly, P., and Ross, C. (2007, August 27). Farming the concrete jungle. *In These Times,* pp. 1–3.

Cooper, A., and Page, A. (2010). Objective measurement of children's physical activity in the environment: UK perspective. In A. A. Lake, T. G. Townshend, and S. Alvanides (Eds.), *Obesogenic environments: Complexities, perceptions, and objective measures* (pp. 81–95). Oxford, UK: Blackwell Publishing.

Cooper, C. (2009a). Fat activism in ten astonishing, beguiling, inspiring, and beautiful episodes. In C. Tomrley and A. K. Naylor (Eds), *Fat studies in the UK.* York: Raw Nerve Books.

Cooper, C. (2009b). *Fat liberation: How fat activism expands the obesity debate.* http://www.charlottecooper.net/downloads/fatstuff/workingpaper_obesityd ebatefactactivism.pdf. Accessed 9/3/10.

Cooper, C. (2010). Fat studies: Mapping the field. *Sociology Compass,* 4, no. 1: 1020–1034.

Cope, M. B., and Allison, D. B. (2010). White hat bias: Examples of its presence in obesity research and a call for renewed commitment to faithfulness in research. *International Journal of Obesity,* 34, no. 1: 84–88.

Corburn, J. (2005). *Street science: Community knowledge and environmental health justice.* Cambridge, MA: MIT Press.

Corburn, J. (2009). *Toward the healthy city: People, places, and the politics of urban planning.* Cambridge, MA: MIT Press.

Corrada, M. M., and Paganini-Hill, A. (2010). Being overweight in adults aged 70–75 is associated with a reduction in mortality risk compared with a normal BMI. *Evidence-Based Medicine.* doi:10.1136/ebm1086.

Correa, N. P., Murray, N. G., Mei, C. A., Baun, W. B., Gor, B. J., Hare, N. B., Banarjee, D., Sindha, M. F., and Jones, L. A. (2010). CAN DO Houston: A community-based approach to preventing childhood obesity. *Preventing Chronic Disease Dialogue,* 7, no. 4: 1–9.

Covington, C. D., King, J. A., Ferrell, I., Jones, C., Hutchinson, C., and Evans, A. (2010). Developing a community-based stroke prevention intensive course in minority communities: The DC Angel Project. *Journal of Neuroscience Nursing*, 42, no. 3: 139–142.

Critser, G. (2003). *Fat land: How Americans became the fattest people in the world.* Boston: Houghton Mifflin.

Crosnoe, R. (2007). Gender, obesity, and education. *Sociology of Education*, 80, no. 3: 241–260.

Crothers, L. M., Kehle, T. J., Bray, M. A., and Theodore, L. A. (2009). Correlates and suspected causes of obesity in children. *Psychology in the Schools*, 46, no. 8: 787–796.

Cruz, T. B., Wright, L. T., and Crawford, G. (2010). The menthol marketing mix: Targeted promotions for focus communities in the United States. *Nicotine and Tobacco Research*, 12, suppl. 2: S147–S153.

Cummings, L. (2003, February 5). The diet business: Banking on failure. *BBC News.* www.http://news.bbc.couk/2/hi/business/2725943.stm. Accessed 7/6/10.

Cummins, S., and Macintyre, S. (2008). Food environments and obesity— neighbourhood or nation? *International Journal of Epidemiology*, 35, no. 1: 100–104.

Currie, J., Della Vigna, S., Moretti, E., and Pathania, V. (2009). The effect of fast food restaurants on obesity and weight gain. *American Economic Journal: Economic Policy*, 2:34–68.

Cut the Waist. (2009). The origins and limitations of BMI. http://www.cutthewaist .com/bmihtml. Accessed 9/1/10.

Cutter, S. (1995). Race, class, and environmental justice. *Progress in Human Geography*, 19, no. 2: 111–122.

Cutts, S. B., Darby, K. J., Boone, C. G., and Brewis, A. (2009). City structure, obesity, and environmental justice: An integrated analysis of physical and social barriers to walkable streets and park access. *Social Science and Medicine*, 69, no. 9: 1314–1322.

Dahmann, N., Walch, J., Joassart-Marcelli, P., Reynolds, K., and Jerrett, M. (2009). The active city? Disparities in provision of urban public recreational resources. *Health and Place*, 16, no. 3: 431–445.

Dant, R. P. (2008). A futuristic research agenda for the field of franchising. *Journal of Small Business Management*, 46, no. 1: 91–98.

DasGupta, S., Fornari, A., Geer, K., Hahn, L., Kumar, V., Lee, H. J., Rubin, S., and Gold, M. (2006). Medical education for social justice: Paulo Freire revisited. *Journal of Medical Humanity*, 27, no. 4: 245–251.

Dave, J. M., An, L. C., Jeffery, R. W., and Ahluwalia, J. S. (2009). Relationship of attitudes toward fast food and frequency of fast-food intake in adults. *Obesity*, 17, no. 6: 1164–1170.

Davidson, M., and Knafl, K. A. (2006). Dimensional analysis of the concept of obesity. *Journal of Advanced Nursing*, 54, no. 3: 342–350.

Davis, J. D., Johnston, L. D., and O'Malley, P. M. (2007). The epidemiology of over-weight and related lifestyle behaviors: Racial/ethnic and socioeconomic status differences among American youth. *American Journal of Preventive Medicine,* 33, no. 4, suppl. 1: S178–S186.

Day, K. (2006). Active living and social justice: Planning for physical activity in low-income, Black, and Latino communities. *Journal of the American Planning Association,* 72, no. 1: 88–97.

Day, K., Boarnet, M., Alfonzo, M., and Forsyth, A. (2006). The Irvine-Minnesota Inventory to Measure Built Environments: Development. *American Journal of Preventive Medicine,* 30, no. 2: 144–152.

Dayton, L., Sharfstein, J., and Hamburg, M. (2010). Tobacco product regulation—A public health approach. *New England Journal of Medicine,* 362:1753–1756.

De Jesus, M. (2009). The importance of social context in understanding and pro-moting low-income immigrant women's health. *Journal of Health Care for the Poor and Underserved,* 20, no. 1: 90–97.

De la Salle, J., and Holland, M. (2010). *Agricultural urbanism: Handbook for building sustainable food systems in 21st century cities.* Winnipeg, Manitoba, Canada: Green Frigate Books.

Delgado, M. (1999). *Social work practice in nontraditional urban settings.* New York: Oxford University Press.

Delgado, M. (2000). *Community social work practice in an urban context: The potential of a capacity-enhancement perspective.* New York: Oxford University Press.

Delgado, M. (2006). *Designs and methods for youth-led research.* Thousand Oaks, CA: Sage Publications.

Delgado, M. (2007). *Social work practice with Latinos: A cultural assets paradigm.* New York: Oxford University Press.

Delgado, M. (2009). *Older adult–led health promotion in urban communities: Theory and models.* Lanham, MD: Rowman and Littlefield.

Delgado, M. (2011). *Latino small businesses and the American dream: Community social work and economic and social development.* New York: Columbia University Press.

Delgado, M., and Humm-Delgado, D. (2009). *Health and health care in the nation's prisons: Issues, challenges, and policies.* Lanham, MD: Rowman and Littlefield.

Delgado, M., and Humm-Delgado, D. (in press). *Asset assessment and community social work practice.* New York: Oxford University Press.

Delgado, M., and Staples, L. (2008). *Youth-led community organizing: Theory and action.* New York: Oxford University Press.

Delgado, M., and Zhou, H. (2008). *Youth-led health promotion in urban communities: A community capacity-enhancement perspective.* Lanham, MD: Rowman and Littlefield.

Delva, J., Johnston, L. D., and O'Malley, P. M. (2007). The epidemiology of over-weight and related lifestyle behaviors: Racial/ethnic and socioeconomic status differences among American youth. *American Journal of Preventive Medicine,* 33, no. 4, suppl. 1: S178–S186.

DeMattia, L., and Denney, S. L. (2008). Childhood obesity prevention: Successful community-based efforts. *Annals of the American Academy of Political and Social Sciences,* 615, no. 1: 83–99.

Denison, D. C. (2010, October 19). Rich produce at city's farmers markets. *Boston Globe,* pp. B1, B11.

Derenne, J. L., and Beresin, E. V. (2006). Body image, media, and eating disorders. *American Journal of Psychiatry,* 30, no. 4: 257–261.

Despommier, D. (2010). *The vertical farm: Feeding the world in the 21st century.* New York: St. Martin's Press.

De Wil, L., Luppino, F., van Straten, A., Penninx, B., Zitman, F., and Cuijpers, P. (2010). Depression and obesity: A meta-analysis of community-based studies. *Psychiatry Research,* 178, no. 2: 230–235.

Dietz, W. H. (2006). Government perspective. In Institute of Medicine, *Perspectives on the prevention of childhood obesity in children and youth* (pp. 33–39). Washington, DC: National Academies Press.

Dietz, W. H., Story, M. T., and Leviton, L. C. (2009). Issues and implications of screening, surveillance, and reporting of children's BMI. *Pediatrics,* 124:98–101.

Dijkum, C. (2000). A methodology for conducting interdisciplinary social research. *European Journal of Operational Research,* 128, no. 2: 290–299.

Dikec, M. (2001). Justice and the spatial imagination. *Environment and Planning,* 33, no. 3: 1785–1805.

Dillard, J. M. (2008). Sloop Jo, slop, Sloppy Joe: How USDA commodities dumping ruined the National School Lunch Program. *Oregon Law Review,* 87:221–258.

Dinour, L. M., Bergen, D., and Yeh, M. C. (2007). The food insecurity–obesity paradox: A review of the literature and the role food stamps may play. *Journal of the American Dietetic Association,* 107, no. 11: 1952–1961.

Donald, B., Gertler, M., Gray, M., and Lobao, L. (2010). Regionalizing the food system? *Cambridge Journal of Regions, Economy, and Society,* 3, no. 2: 171–175.

Donaldson, L. P., and Daughtery, L. C. (2011). Introducing asset-based models of social justice into service learning: A social work approach. *Journal of Community Practice,* 19, no. 1: 80–99.

Dorfman, L., and Wallack, L. (2007). Moving nutrition upstream: The case for reframing obesity. *Journal of Nutrition Education and Behavior,* 39, no. 2: S45–S50.

Douglas, S., and Jacobson, M. F. (2010, April 6). Is a soda tax a good policy to reduce obesity in the U.S.? *Atlanta Journal-Constitution,* p. A11.

Dowler, E. (2008). Food and health inequalities: The challenge for sustaining just consumption. *Local Environment: The International Journal of Justice and Sustainability,* 13, no. 8: 759–772.

Drewnowski, A. (2004). Obesity and the food environment: Dietary energy density and diet costs. *American Journal of Preventive Medicine,* 27, no. 3: 154–162.

Drewnowski, A. (2009). Obesity, diet, and social inequalities. *Nutrition Review*, 67, suppl. 1: S36–S39.

Drewnowski, A., Rehm, C. D., and Solet, D. (2007). Disparities in obesity rates: Analysis by ZIP code area. *Social Science and Medicine*, 65, no. 12: 2458–2463.

Drewnowski, A., and Specter, S. E. (2004). Poverty and obesity: The role of energy density and energy costs. *American Journal of Clinical Nutrition*, 79, no. 1: 6–16.

Drummond, R. L., Staten, L. K., Sanford, M. R., Davidson, C. L., Ciocason, M. M., Khor, K.-N., and Kaplan, F. (2009). Step to a Healthier Arizona: A pebble in the pond: The ripple effect of an obesity prevention intervention targeting the child care environment. *Health Promotion Practice*, 10, suppl. 2: 156S–157S.

Duke, R. B. (2010, June 16). Epidemic growth of the Net porn cited: Kids' "innocence at risk." *Washington Times*, p. 4.

Durden, E. D., House, D., Ben-Joseph, R., and Chu, B.-C. (2008). Economic costs of obesity to self-insured employers. *Journal of Occupational and Environmental Medicine*, 50, no. 9: 991–997.

Ebi, K. L. (2009). Environmental justice: Facilitating climate justice through community-based adaptation in the health sector. *Environmental Justice*, 2, no. 4: 191–195.

Ebrahim, S. (2006). Editor's Choice: Obesity, fat, and public health. *International Journal of Epidemiology*, 35, no. 1: 1–2.

Edwards, K. L. (2010). Defining and mapping obesogenic environments for children. In A. A. Lake, T. G. Townshend, and S. Alvanides (Eds.), *Obesogenic environments: Complexities, perceptions, and objective measures* (pp. 63–79). Oxford, UK: Blackwell Publishing.

Eid, J., Overman, H. G., Puga, D., and Turner, M. A. (2008). Fat city: Questioning the relationship between urban sprawl and obesity. *Journal of Urban Economics*, 63, no. 2: 385–404.

Eitzen, D. S., and Stewart, K. (Eds.). (2007). *Solutions to social problems: From the bottom up: Successful social movements*. Boston: Pearson Publishers.

Elias, M. (2002, April 30). Hospital tab for obese kids: $127M a year. *USA Today*, p. 1.

Elliott, P. T. (2010). Individual and socio-environmental determinants of overweight and obesity in urban Canada. *Health Place*, 16, no. 2: 389–398.

Elliott, S. (2011, April 5). A growing population, and target, for marketers. *New York Times*, p. B2.

Engelhard, C. L., Garson, A., and Dorn, S. (2009). Reducing obesity: Policy strategies from the tobacco wars. *Methodist DeBakey Cardiovascular Journal*, 5, no. 4: 46–50.

Epstein, L. H., Beecher, M. D., Beecher, B. S., Graf, J. L., and Roemmich, J. N. (2007). Choice of interactive dance and bicycle games in overweight and nonoverweight youth. *Annals of Behavioral Medicine*, 33, no. 2: 124–131.

Estarziau, M., Morales, M., Rico, A., Margellos-Anast, H., Whitman, S., and Christoffel, K. K. (2006). *The community survey in Humboldt Park: Preventing obesity and improving health*. Chicago: Sinai Urban Health Institute.

Ethan, M., Berke, E. M., Koepsell, T. D., Moudon, A. V., Hoskins, R. E., and Larson, E. B. (2007). Association of the built environment with physical activity and obesity in older persons. *American Journal of Public Health*, 97, no. 3: 486–492.

European Union Public Health System. (2009). *Overweight: Limitations of BMI as a measure of overweight and obesity*. hhp://www.euphix.org/object_document/04852n27195.html. Accessed 8/31/10.

Evangelista, A. N., Ortiz, A. R., Rios-Soto, K. R., and Urdapilleta, A. (2004). *U.S.A. the fast food nation: Obesity as an epidemic*. Tempe: Arizona State University, Department of Mathematics and Statistics.

Evans, B., and Colls, R. (2009). Measuring fatness, governing bodies: The spatialities of the Body Mass Index (BMI) in anti-obesity politics. *Antipode*, 41, no. 5: 1051–1083.

Evans, J., Rich, E., Davies, B., and Allwood, R. (2008). *Education, disordered eating, and obesity discourses: Fat fabrications*. London: Routledge.

Everett, M., Mejia, A., and Quiroz, O. (2009). Building evidence to prevent childhood obesity: Lessons from the Portland Healthy Eating Active Living (HEAL) Coalition. *Practicing Anthropology*, 31, no. 4: 21–26.

Ewing, R. (2005). Building environment to promote health. *Journal of Epidemiology and Community Health*, 69, no. 10: 536–537.

Ewing, R., Schmid, T., Killingsworth, R., Zlot, A., and Raudenbush, S. (2008). Relationship between urban sprawl and physical activity, obesity, and morbidity. In J. Marzluff, E. Shulenberger, W. Endlicher, M. Alberti, G. Bradley, C. Ryan, U. Simon, and C. ZumBrunnen (Eds.), *Urban ecology: An international perspective on the interaction between humans and nature* (pp. 567–582). New York: Springer.

Esparza, L. A., Morales-Campos, D. Y., Mojica, C. M., and Parra-Medina, D. (2010). Engaging Latino adolescent girls in physical activity intervention planning in a low-income, urban environment. Texas Obesity Research Center. *International Journal of Exercise Science: Conference Abstract Submissions*, vol. 6, lss 1, article 38.

Ezzati, M., Martin, H., Skjold, S., Hoom, S. V., and Murray, C. J. L. (2006). Trends in national and state-level obesity in the USA after corrections for self-report bias: Analysis of health survey. *JRSM*, 99, no. 5: 250–257.

Faber, D. (1998). The struggle for ecological democracy and environmental justice. In D. Faber (Ed.), *The struggle for ecological democracy: Environmental justice movements in the United States* (pp. 1–26). New York: Guilford Press.

Fainstein, S. S. (2008). *Spatial justice and planning*. Paper presented at the International Conference Justice Spatiale: Spatial Justice, Nanterre.

Fainstein, S. S. (2010). *The just city*. Ithaca, NY: Cornell University Press.

Fam, D., Mosley, E., Lopes, A., Mathieson, L., Morison, J., and Connellan, G. (2008). *Irrigation of urban green spaces: A review of the environmental, social, and economic benefits*. Technical report no. 04/08. Australia: Cooperative Research Centre for Irrigation Futures.

Farley, T., and Daines, R. F. (2010, October 7). No food stamps for sodas. *New York Times*, p. A26.

Feenstra, G. W. (1997). Local food systems and sustainable communities. *American Journal of Alternative Agriculture*, 12, no. 1: 28–36.

Ferguson, R. (2007). *Obesity: As it is experienced in the United States, Massachusetts, and Boston, and effective strategies to confront the epidemic.* http://www.fergsfitness.com/obesity.htm. Accessed 7/27/10.

Fetterman, D. M., and Wandersman, A. (Eds.). (2004). *Empowerment evaluation principles in practice.* New York: Guilford Press.

Field, A. E. (2007a). Obesity prevention during preschool and elementary school-age years. In S. Kumanyika and R. C. Brownson (Eds.), *Handbook of obesity prevention: A resource for health professionals* (pp. 429–454). New York: Springer.

Field, A. E. (2007b). Obesity prevention during preadolescence and adolescence. In S. Kumanyika and R. C. Brownson (Eds.), *Handbook of obesity prevention: A resource for health professionals* (pp. 459–488). New York: Springer.

Findholt, N. E., Michael, Y. L., Davis, M. M., and Brogetti, V. W. (2010). Environmental influences on children's physical activity and diets in rural Oregon: Results of a youth photovoice project. *Online Journal of Rural Nursing and Health Care*, 10, 2.

Finkelstein, E. A., Fiebelkorn, F. E., and Wang, G. (2005). The costs of obesity among full-time employees. *American Journal of Health Promotion*, 20, no. 1: 45–51.

Finkelstein, E. A., Trogdon, J. G., Cohen, J. W., and Dietz, W. (2009). Annual medical spending attributable to obesity: Payer- and service-specific estimates. *Health Affairs*, 28, no. 5: w822–w831.

Finkelstein, E. A., and Zuckerman, L. (2008). *The fattening of America: How the economy makes us fat, if it matters, and what to do about it.* New York: John Wiley.

Finster, M. E., Gray, K. A., and Binns, H. J. (2004). Lead levels of edibles grown in contaminated residential soils: A field survey. *Science of the Total Environment*, 320:245–257.

Fisher, D. M. W. (2010). *An inquiry to explore significant regional obesity prevalence factors in the United States.* UMI ProQuest Dissertations and Theses.

Fitzgibbon, M. L., Stolley, M. R., Schiffer, L., Horn, L. V., Christoffel, K. K., and Dyer, A. (2005). Two-year follow-up results for Hip-Hop to Health Jr.: A randomized controlled trial for overweight prevention in preschool minority children. *Journal of Pediatrics*, 146, no. 5: 618–625.

Fitzpatrick, K., and LaGory, M. (2000). *Unhealthy places: The ecology of risk in the urban landscape.* New York: Routledge.

Flegal, K. M. (2005). Epidemiologic aspects of overweight and obesity in the United States. *Physiology and Behavior*, 86, no. 5: 599–602.

Flegal, K. M. (2006). Commentary: The epidemic of obesity—What's in a name? *International Journal of Epidemiology*, 35, no. 1: 72–77.

Flegal, K. M., Carroll, M. D., Ogden, C. L., and Curtin, L. R. (2010). Prevalence and trends in obesity among US adults, 1999–2008. *Journal of the American Medical Association*, 303, no. 3: 235–241.

Flegal, K. M., and Ogden, C. L. (2011). Childhood obesity: Are we all speaking the same language? *Advances in Nutrition: An International Review Journal*, 2, no. 1: 1595–1665.

Flegal, K. M., Williamson, D. F., Pamuk, E. R., and Rosenberg, H. M. (2004). Estimating deaths attributable to obesity in the United States. *American Journal of Public Health*, 94, no. 9: 1486–1489.

Flegal, K. M., et al. (2009). Comparisons of body fat, body mass index, waist circumference, and waist-stature ratio in adults. *American Journal of Clinical Nutrition*, 89, no. 2: 500–508.

Fletcher, A., and Vaurus, J. (2006). *The guide to social change led by and with young people*. Olympia, WA: CommonAction.

Flicker, L., McCaul, K. A., Hankey, G. J., Brown, W. J., Byles, J. E., and Almeida. O. P. (2010). Body mass index and survival in men and women aged 70–75. *Journal of the American Geriatrics Society*, 58, no. 2: 234–241.

Flores, G. R. (2008). Active living in Latino communities. *American Journal of Preventive Medicine*, 34, no. 4: 369–370.

Flores, K. S. (2008). *Youth participatory evaluation: Strategies for engaging young people*. San Francisco: Jossey-Bass.

Flores, R. (1995). Dance for health: Improving fitness in African American and Hispanic adolescents. *Public Health Reports*, 110, no. 2: 189–193.

Flores-Gonzalez, N., Rodriguez, M., and Rodriguez-Muniz, M. (2006). From hip-hop to humanization: Batey Urbano as a space for Latino youth culture and community action. In S. Ginwright, P. Noguera, and J. Cammarota (Eds.), *Beyond resistance: Youth activism and community change* (pp. 175–196). New York: Routledge.

Fogli, J. J. (2005). Measuring body composition: Keeping up with an increasingly obese population. *Obesity Research*, 13:1134.

Ford, E. G., Veur, S. S. V., and Foster, G. D. (2007). Obesity prevention in school and group child care settings. In S. Kumanyika and R. C. Brownson (Eds.), *Handbook of obesity prevention: A resource for health professionals* (pp. 349–376). New York: Springer.

Foresight. (2007). *Tackling obesity: Future Choices—Project Report* (2nd ed.). London: Government Office of Science. http://www.foresight.gov.uk. Accessed 10/13/10.

Foster, G. D., Borradile, K. E., Grundy, K. M., Veur, S. S. V., Nachmani, J., Karpyn, A., Kumanyika, S., and Shults, J. (2008). A policy-based school intervention to prevent overweight and obesity. *Pediatrics*, 121, no. 4: e794–e802.

Francoeur, R., and Elkins, J. (2006). Older adults with diabetes and complications. In B. Berkman and S. D'Ambruoso (Eds.), *Handbook of social work in health and aging* (pp. 29–40). New York: Oxford University Press.

Frank, J., and Di Ruggiero, E. (2003). Prevention: Delivering the goods. *Hospital Quarterly*, 6, no. 3: suppl. 2–8.

Frank, L. D., Andresen, M. A., and Schmid, T. L. (2004). Obesity relationships with community design, physical activity, and time spent in cars. *American Journal of Preventive Medicine*, 27, no. 1: 87–96.

Frank, L. D., and Engelke, P. O. (2001). The built environment and human activity patterns: Exploring the impacts of urban form on public health. *Journal of Planning Literature*, 19, no. 2: 202–218.

Freedman, D. A. (2009). Local food environments: They're all stocked differently. *American Journal of Community Psychology*, 44, no. 4: 382–393.

Freeman, A. (2007). Fast food: Oppression through poor nutrition. *California Law Review*, 95:2221–2259.

Freudenberg, N., Bradley, S. P., and Serrano, M. (2009). Public health campaigns to change industry practices that damage health: An analysis of 12 case studies. *Health Education and Behavior*, 36, no. 2: 230–249.

Freudenberg, N., and Galea, S. (2010). Cities of consumption: The impact of corporate practices on health or urban populations. *Journal of Urban Health*, 85, no. 4: 462–471.

Friedman, R. R. (2005). *Community action to change school food policy: An organizing kit*. Boston: Massachusetts Public Health Association.

Frumkin, H. (2002). Urban sprawl and public health. *Public Health Reports*, 117, no. 2: 201–217.

Galvez, M. P., Hong, B. B., Choi, E., Liao, L., Godbold, J., and Brenner, B. (2009). Childhood obesity and neighborhood food-store availability in an inner-city community. *Academic Pediatrics*, 9, no. 5: 339–343.

Galvez, M. P., Morland, K., Raines, C., Kobil, J., Siskind, J., Godbold, J., and Breener, B. (2008). Race and food store availability in an inner-city neighborhood. *Public Health Nutrition*, 11, no. 6: 624–631.

Garcia, R., and Fenwick, C. (2008). Social science, equal justice, and public health policy: Lessons from Los Angeles. *Journal of Public Health Policy*, 30, suppl.: S26–S32.

Gard, M., and Wright, J. (2005). *The obesity epidemic: Science, morality, and ideology*. New York: Routledge.

Geana, M. V., Kimminau, K. S., and Greiner, K. A. (2011). Sources of information in a multiethnic, underserved, urban community: Does ethnicity matter? *Journal of Communication: International Perspectives*, 16, no. 6: 583–594.

Gee, G. C., Ro, A., Garvin, A., and Takeuchi, D. T. (2008). Disentangling the effects of racial and weight discrimination on body mass index and obesity among Asian Americans. *American Journal of Public Health*, 98, no. 3: 493–500.

Ghirardelli, A., Quinn, V., and Foerster, S. B. (2010). Using geographic information systems and local food store data in California's low-income neighborhoods to inform community initiatives and resources. *American Journal of Public Health*, 100, no. 11: 2156–2162.

Gibbs, W. W. (2005). Obesity: An overblown epidemic? *Scientific American*, 292, no. 6: 70–77.

Gibson, D. (2003). Food stamp program participation is positively related to obesity in low income women. *Journal of Nutrition*, 133, no. 7: 2225–2231.

Giles-Corti, B. (2006). People or places: What should be the target? *Patient Education and Counseling*, 9, no. 5: 357–366.

Gilman, S. L. (2008). *Fat: A cultural history of obesity*. Malden, MA: Polity Press.

Gilman, S. L. (2010). *Obesity: The biography*. New York: Oxford University Press.

Glassman, M. E., Figueroa, M., and Irigoyen, M. (2011). Latino parents' perceptions of their ability to prevent obesity in their children. *Family and Community Health*, 34, no. 1: 4–16.

Glazer, S. (2007). Slow food movement: Can it change eating habits? *Congressional Quarterly Researcher*, 17, no. 4: 1–31.

Gob, Y.-Y., Bogart, L. M., Sipple-Asher, B. K., Uyeda, K., Hawes-Dawson, J., Olarita-Dhungana, J., Ryan, G. W., and Schuster, M. A. (2009). Using community-based participatory research to identify potential interventions to overcome barriers to adolescents' healthy eating and physical activity. *Journal of Behavioral Medicine*, 32, no. 4: 491–502.

Golub, M., Charlop, M., Groisman-Perelstein, A. E., Ruddock, C., and Calman, N. (2011). Got low-fat milk? How a community-based coalition changed school milk policy in New York City. *Family and Community Health*, 34, suppl.: S44–S53.

Goodman, M. K. (2009). Contemporary food matters? A review essay. *International Planning Studies*, 14, no. 4: 437–442.

Gorber, S. C., Treblay, M., Moher, D., and Gorber, B. (2006) A comparison of direct vs. self-report measures for assessing height, weight, and body mass index: A systematic review. *Obesity Reviews*, 8, no. 4: 307–326.

Gordon, H. R. (2010). *We fight to win: Inequality and the politics of youth activism.* New Brunswick, NJ: Rutgers University Press.

Gordon-Larsen, P., Nelson, M. C., Page, P., and Popkins, B. M. (2006). Inequality in the built environment underlies key health disparities in physical activity and obesity. *Pediatrics*, 117, no. 2: 417–424.

Goren, A., Harris, J. L., Schwartz, M. B., and Brownell, K. D. (2010). Predicting support for restricting food marketing to youth. *Health Affairs*, 29, no. 3: 419–424.

Gostin, L. O. (2007). Law as a tool to facilitate healthier lifestyles and prevent obesity. *Journal of the American Medical Association*, 297, no. 1: 87–90.

Gottlieb, R. (2009). Where we live, work, play . . . and eat: Expanding the environmental justice agenda. *Environmental Justice*, 2, no. 1: 7–8.

Gottlieb, R., and Fisher, A. (1996). "First feed the face": Environmental justice and community food security. *Antipode*, 28, no. 2: 193–203.

Gottlieb, R., and Joshi, A. (2010). *Food justice*. Cambridge, MA: MIT Press.

Government Accountability Office. (2009, June 30). *U.S. Agriculture: Retail food prices grew faster than the prices farmers received for agricultural commodities, but economic research has not established that concentration has affected these trends.* (09–746R). Washington, DC: Author.

Grabe, S., Ward, L. M., and Hyde, J. S. (2008). The role of the media in body image concerns among women: A meta-analysis of experimental and correlational studies. *Psychological Bulletin*, 134, no. 3: 460–476.

Grady, D. (2010, August 4). Obesity rates keep rising, troubling health officials. *New York Times*, p. A11.

Graf, S., and Ackerman, J. (2009). A special role for lawyers in a social norm change movement: From tobacco control to childhood obesity prevention. *Preventing Chronic Disease*, 6, no. 3: A95–A100.

Granner, M. L., and Sharpe, P. A. (2004). Evaluation of community coalition characteristics and functioning: A survey of measurement tools. *Health Education Research*, 19, no. 5: 514–532.

Gray, J. *BMI, social justice, and community gardens.* Unpublished manuscript, Boston University School of Social Work.

Green, M. (2007). Oakland looks towards greener pastures: The Oakland Food Policy Council. *Edible East Bay*, 36–37.

Greenblatt, A. (2003). Obesity epidemic: Can Americans change their self-destructive habits? *Congressional Quarterly Researcher*, 13, no. 4: 1–41.

Greenfield, K. T. (2011, May 15). Taco Bell and the golden age of drive-thru. *Bloomberg Business Week*.

Greer, G. (1971). *The female eunuch.* New York: Harper Perennial.

Grier, S. A., and Kumanyika, S. K. (2008). The context for choice: Health implications of targeted food and beverage marketing to African Americans. *American Journal of Public Health*, 98, no. 9: 1616–1629.

Grier, S. A., and Kumanyika, S. K. (2010). Targeted marketing and public health. *Annual Review of Public Health*, 31:349–369.

Griffith, M. W. (2003, December 25). The "Food Justice" Movement: Trying to break the food chains. *Black Commentator*, issue 70. www.BlackCommentator.com. Accessed 7/16/10.

Groessl, E. J., Kaplan, R. M., Barrett-Connor, E., and Ganials, T. G. (2004). Body mass indexed quality of well-being in a community of older adults. *American Journal of Preventive Medicine*, 26, no. 2: 126–129.

Grol-Prokocpczyk, H. (2009). *WHO says obesity is an epidemic? How excess weight became an American crisis.* Paper presented at the annual meeting of the American Sociological Association, Philadelphia.

Gross, J. E. (2006–2007). The First Amendment and diet industry advertisement: How puffery in weight-loss advertisements has gone too far. *Journal of Law and Health*, 20:325–356.

Grow, H. M., Cook, A. J., Arterburn, D. E., Saelens, B. E., Drewnowski, A., and Lozano, P. (2010). Child obesity associated with social disadvantage of children's neighborhoods. *Social Science and Medicine*, 71, no. 3: 584–591.

Grow, H. M. G., and Saelens, B. E. (2010). Physical activity and environments which promote active living in youth (US). In A. A. Lake, T. G. Townshend, and S. Alvanides (Eds.), *Obesogenic environments: Complexities, perceptions, and objective measures* (pp. 97–115). Oxford, UK: Blackwell Publishing.

Guendelman, M., Cheryan, S., and Monin, B. (2011). Fitting in but getting fat: Identity threat and dietary choices among U.S. immigrant groups. *Psychological Science*, 22, no. 7: 959–967.

Guthman, J. (2007). *Agrarian dream: The paradox of organic farming in California*. Berkeley: University of California Press.

Guthman, J. (2008). Bringing good food to others: Investigating the subjects of alternative food practices. *Cultural Geographies*, 15, no. 4: 431–447.

Hacker, G. A., Collins, R., and Jacobson, M. (1987). *Marketing booze to blacks*. Washington, DC: Center for Science in the Public Interest.

Haines, J., and Neumark-Sztainer, D. (2006). Prevention of obesity and eating disorders: A consideration of shared risk factors. *Health Education Research*, 21, no. 6: 770–782.

Haire-Joshu, D., Fleming, C., and Schermbeck, R. (2007). The role of government in preventing obesity. In S. Kumanyika and R. C. Brownson (Eds.), *Handbook of obesity prevention: A resource for health professionals* (pp. 129–170). New York: Springer.

Haire-Joshu, D., Nanney, M. S., Elliott, M., Davey, C., Caito, N., Loman, D., Brownson, R. C., and Kreuter, M. W. (2010). The use of mentoring programs to improve energy balance behaviors in high-risk children. *Obesity*, 18, suppl.: S75–S83.

Hamm, M. W., and Bellows, A. C. (2003). Community food security and nutrition educators. *Journal of Nutrition Education and Behavior*, 35, no. 1: 37–43.

Hamlin, C. (2008). Is all justice environmental? *Environmental Justice*, 1, no. 3: 145–148.

Hammond, R. A. (2009). Complex systems modeling for obesity research. *Preventing chronic diseases: Public health research, practice, and policy*, 6, no. 3: 1–10.

Handy, S., and Clifton, K. (2007). Planning and the built environment: Implications for obesity prevention. In S. Kumanyika and R. C. Brownson (Eds.), *Handbook of obesity prevention: A resource for health professionals* (pp. 171–192). New York: Springer.

Hansen, Y. (2008). *Food and social justice in Saskatchewan: Community gardens as a local practice of food sovereignty*. Canada: University of Regina.

Harding, A. K., and Holdren, G. R. (1993). Environmental equity and the environmental professional. *Environment Science and Technology*, 27, no. 10: 1990–1993.

Harnack, L., Walters, S., and Jacobs, D. (2002). Dietary intake and food sources of whole grains among U.S. children and adolescents: Where do youths stand in comparison with the *Healthy People* 2010 objectives? *American Journal of Public Health*, 92, no. 10: 844–851.

Harper, A., Shattuck, A., Holt-Giménez, E., Alkon, A., and Lambrick, F. (2009). *Food Policy Councils: Lessons learned*. Oakland, CA: Food First/Institute for Food and Development Policy.

Harrington, D. W., and Elliott, S. J. (2009). Weighing the importance of neighbourhood: A multilevel exploration of the determinants of overweight and obesity. *Social Science and Medicine*, 68, no. 4: 593–600.

Harris, J. L., Brownell, K. D., and Bargh, J. A. (2009). The food marketing defense model: Integrating psychological research to protect youth and inform public policy. *Social Issues and Policy Review*, 3, no. 1: 211–271.

Harris, N., and Hooper, A. (2004). Rediscovering the "spatial" in public policy and planning: An examination of the spatial content of sectoral policy documents. *Planning Theory and Practice*, 5, no. 2: 147–169.

Harrison, J. (2008). Lessons learned from pesticide drift: A call to bring production agriculture, farm labor, and social justice back into agrifood research and activism. *Agriculture and Human Values*, 25, no. 2: 163–167.

Hartocollis, A. (2010, July 2). Failure of state soda tax plan reflects power of an antitax message. *New York Times*, p. A18.

Hartocollis, A. (2011, March 8). Diet plan with hormones has fans and skeptics. *New York Times*, pp. A1, A21.

Harvey, D. (2009). *Social justice and the city* (Rev. ed.). Athens: University of Georgia Press.

Hawken, P. (2007). *Blessed unrest: How the largest movement in the world came into being and why no one saw it coming*. New York: Viking.

Hawn, C. (2009). Take two aspirin and tweet me in the morning: How Twitter, Facebook, and other social media are reshaping health care. *Health Affairs*, 28, no. 2: 361–368.

Hay, A. M. (1995). Concepts of equity, fairness, and justice in geographical studies. *Transactions of the Institute of British Geographers*, New Series, 20: 500–508.

Hayes-Bautista, D. E. (2002). The Latino health research agenda for the twenty-first century. In M. M. Suárez-Orozco and M. M. Páez (Eds.), *Latinos remaking America* (pp. 213–235). Los Angeles: University of California Press.

Health Canada. Division of Childhood and Adolescence. (2002). *Natural and built environments*. Ottawa: Author. http://www.hc-sc.gc.ca/dca-dea/publications/healthy_dev_partb_5_e.html. Accessed 10/15/10.

Hellerstein, D. J., Almeida, G., Devlin, M. J., Mendelsohn, N., Helfand, S., Dragatsi, D., Miranda, R., Kelso, J. R., and Capitelli, L. (2007). Assessing obesity and other related health problems of mentally ill Hispanic patients in an urban outpatient setting. *Psychiatric Quarterly*, 78, no. 2: 171–181.

Hellmich, N. (2003, May 14). An overweight America comes with a hefty price tag. *USA Today*, p. 1.

Helm, S., Stang, J., and Ireland, M. (2009). A garden pilot project enhances fruit and vegetable consumption among children. *Journal of the American Dietetic Association*, 109, no. 7: 1220–1226.

Hendricks, K., Briefel, R., Novak, T., and Ziegler, P. (2006). Maternal and child characteristics associated with infant and toddler feeding practices. *Journal of the American Dietary Association*, 106, suppl. 1: S135–S148.

Hennessy, E., Kraak, V. I., Hyatt, R. R., Bloom, J., Fenton, M., Wagoner, C., and Economos, C. D. (2010). Active living for rural children: Community perspectives using PhotoVOICE. *American Journal of Preventive Medicine*, 39, no. 6: 537–545.

Herndon, A. M. (2010). Mommy made me do it: Mothering fat children in the midst of the obesity epidemic. *Food, Culture, and Society: An International Journal of Multidisciplinary Research*, 13, no. 3: 331–349.

Hess, D. J. (2009). *Localist movements in a global economy: Sustainability, justice, and urban development in the United States*. Cambridge, MA: MIT Press.

Hesse-Biber, S., Leavy, P., Quinn, C. E., and Zoino, J. (2006). The mass marketing of disordered eating and eating disorders: The social psychology of women, thinness, and culture. *Women's Studies International Forum*, 29:208–224.

Hill, A. J. (2004). Does dieting make you fat? *British Journal of Nutrition*, 92: S15–S18.

Hill, J. O., Wyatt, H. R., Reed, G. W., and Peters, J. C. (2003). Obesity and the environment: Where do we go from here? *Science*, 299, no. 5608: 853–855.

Hillier, A., Cole, B. L., Smith, T. E., Yancey, A. K., Williams, J. D., Grier, S. A., and McCarthy, W. J. (2009). Clustering of unhealthy outdoor advertisements around child-serving institutions: A comparison of three cities. *Health and Place*, 15, no. 4: 935–945.

Himes, J. H. (2009). Challenges of accurately measuring and using BMI and other indicators of obesity in children. *Pediatrics*, 124, no. 1: 3–22.

Hinds, J., and Sparks, P. (2009). Investigating environmental identity, well-being, and meaning. *Ecopsychology*, 1, no. 4: 181–186.

Hinrichs, C. C., and Allen, P. (2008). Selective patronage and social justice: Local food consumer campaigns in historical context. *Journal of Agricultural and Environmental Ethics*, 21, no. 4: 329–352.

Hodge, D. R., Jackson, K. P., and Vaughn, M. G. (2010). Culturally sensitive interventions for health related behaviors among Latino youth: A meta-analytic review. *Children and Youth Services Review*, 32, no. 10: 1331–1337.

Hodge, J. G., Garcia, A. M., and Shah, S. (2008). Legal themes concerning obesity regulations in the United States: Theory and practice. *Australia and New Zealand Health Policy*, 5, no. 1: 5–14.

Hodgson, K. (2009, August/September). Where food planning and health intersect. *Connect*, 1–8.

Hoefer, R. (2006). *Advocacy practice for social justice*. Chicago: Lyceum Books.

Hoff, R., Mahfood, J., and McGuiness, A. (2010). *Sustainable benefits of urban farming as a potential brownfields remedy*. Bridgeville, PA: Mahfood Group.

Hofstader, R. (1964). *Anti-intellectualism in American life*. New York: Alfred A. Knopf.

Holifield, R. (2001). Defining environmental justice and environmental racism. *Urban Geography,* 22: 78–90.

Holt-Giménez, E., and Shattuck, A. (2011). Food crises, food regimes, and food movements: Rumblings of reform or tides of transformation? *Journal of Peasant Studies,* 38, no. 1: 109–144.

Honisett, S., Woolcock, S., Porter, C., and Hughes, I. (2009). Developing an award program for children's settings to supplement eating and physical activity and reduce the risk of overweight and obesity. *BMC Public Health,* 9, no. 10: 345.

Honneth, A. (1995). *The struggle for recognition: The moral grammar of social conflicts.* Cambridge, MA: MIT Press.

Hopkins, P. (2011). Teaching and learning guide for: Critical geographies of body size. *Geography Compass,* 6, no. 2: 106–111.

Horowitz, A. (2006). Overview. In B. Berkman and S. D'Ambruoso (Eds.), *Handbook of social work in health and aging* (pp. 5–6). New York: Oxford University Press.

Hosang, D. (2006). Beyond policy: Ideology, race, and the reimagining of youth. In S. Ginwright, P. Noguera, and J. Cammarota (Eds.), *Beyond resistance: Youth activism and community change* (pp. 3–19). New York: Routledge.

Hosler, A., Varadarajulu, D., Ronsani, A. E., Fredrick, B. L., and Fisher, B. (2006). Low-fat milk and high-fiber bread availability in food stores in urban and rural communities. *Journal of Public Health Management and Practice,* 12, no. 6: 556–562.

Hou, J., Johnson, J. M., and Lawson, L. J. (2009). *Greening cities, growing communities: Learning from Seattle's urban community gardens.* Seattle: University of Washington Press.

Houston Chronicle. (2011, February 18). Food deserts: We need more grocery stores in Houston. And we need them in the right places, p. 1.

Howard, E. (1946). *Garden cities of tomorrow.* London: Faber and Faber.

Howe, L. D., Patel, R., and Galobardes, B. (2010). Commentary. Tipping the balance: Wider waistlines in men but wider inequalities in women. *International Journal of Epidemiology,* 39, no. 2: 404–405.

Hsu, M., Anen, C., and Quartz, S. R. (2008). The right and the good: Distributive justice and neural encoding of equality and efficiency. *Science,* 320, no. 5879: 1092–1096.

Hu, F. B. (2008). *Obesity epidemiology.* New York: Oxford University Press.

Hu, W. (2011, October 4). Schools dangle carrot snacks, but it's a tough sale. *New York Times,* p. A20.

Huang, T.-K., and Glass, T. A. (2008). Transforming research strategies for understanding and preventing obesity. *Journal of the American Medical Association,* 300, no. 15: 1811–1813.

Huberty, J. L., Baluff, M., O'Dell, M., and Peterson, K. (2010). From good ideas to actions. A model driven community collaborative to prevent childhood obesity. *Preventive Medicine,* 50, suppl. 1: S36–S43.

Hung, Y. (2004). East New York farms: Youth participation in community development and urban agriculture. *Children, Youth, and Environments,* 14, no. 1: 20–31.

Hutch, D. J., Bouye, K. E., Skillen, E., Lee, C., Whitehead, L., and Rashid, J. R. (2011). Potential strategies to eliminate built environment disparities for disadvantaged and
vulnerable communities. *American Journal of Public Health,* 101, no. 4: 587–595.

Hyde, R. (2008). Europe battles with obesity. *The Lancet,* 371, no. 9631: 2160–2161.

Hynes, H. P. (1995). *A patch of Eden: America's inner-city gardeners.* White River
Junction, VT: Chelsea Green.

Hynes, H. P., and Howe, G. (2002). *Urban horticulture in the contemporary United
States: Personal and community benefits.* Paper presented at the International
Conference on Urban Horticulture, Wadenswil, Switzerland.

Inagmi, S., Cohen, D. A., Brown, A. R., and Asch, S. M. (2009). Body mass index,
neighborhood fast food and restaurant concentration, and car ownership. *Journal of Urban Health,* 86, no. 5: 683–695.

Innes, S. (2010, June 30). Date: 33% of Arizona Hispanics are obese. *Arizona Daily
Star,* p. A1.

Irigoyen, M., Glassman, M. E., Chen, S., and Findley, S. E. (2008). Early onset of
overweight and obesity among low-income 1- to 5-year olds in New York City.
Journal of Urban Health, 85, no. 4: 545–554.

Irons, M. E. (2010, November 16). City wants to plow vacant plots to farm land.
Boston Globe, pp. B1, B6.

Isganaitis, E., and Levitsky, L. L. (2008). Preventing childhood obesity: Can we do it?
Current Opinion in Endocrinology, Diabetes, and Obesity, 15, no. 1: 1–8.

Israel, B. A., Krieger, J., Vlahov, D., Ciske, S., Foley, M., Fortin, P., Guzman, J. R.,
Lichtenstein, R., McGranaghan, R., Palermo, A., and Tang, G. (2006). Challenges
and facilitating factors in sustaining community-based participatory research
partnerships: Lessons learned from the Detroit, New York City, and Seattle Urban Research Centers. *Journal of Urban Health,* 83, no. 6: 1022–1040.

Ivanova, L., Dimitrov, P., Dellava, J., and Hoffman, D. (2008). Prevalence of obesity and overweight among urban adults in Bulgaria. *Public Health Nutrition,* 11,
no. 12: 1407–1410.

Jabs, J., and Devine, C. M. (2006). Time scarcity and food choices: An overview.
Appetite, 47, no. 2: 196–204.

Jackson, C. J., Mullis, R. M., and Hughes, M. (2010). Development of a theatre-
based nutrition and physical activity intervention for low-income, urban, African
American adolescents. *Progress in Community Health Partnerships: Research,
Education, and Action,* 4, no. 2: 89–98.

Jacobson, P. L., Racioppi, F., and Rutter, H. (2009). Who owns the roads? How mo-
torized traffic discourages walking and bicycling. *Injury Prevention,* 15, no. 2:
369–373.

James, K. S., Connelly, C. D., Rutkowski, E., McPherson, D., Garcia, L., Mareno, N.,
and Zinkle, D. (2008). Family-based weight management with Latino mothers
and children. *Journal of Specialists in Pediatric Nursing,* 13, no. 4: 249–262.

James, W. P. T. (2008). The epidemiology of obesity: The size of the problem. *Journal of Internal Medicine*, 263, no. 4: 336–352.

James, W. P. T., Jackson-Leach, R., and Rigby, N. (2010). An international perspective on obesity and obesogenic environments. In A. A. Lake, T. G. Townshend, and S. Alvanides (Eds.), *Obesogenic environments: Complexities, perceptions, and objective measures* (pp. 1–9). Oxford, UK: Blackwell Publishing.

Janssen, I., and Mark, A. E. (2007). Elevated body mass index and mortality risk in the elderly. *Obesity Reviews*, 8, no. 1: 41–59.

Jebb, S. A., and Prentice, A. M. (2001). Single definition of overweight and obesity should be used. *British Medical Journal*, 323, no. 7319: 999.

Johnson, C. (2010). The magic of group identity: How predatory lenders use minorities to target communities of color. *Georgetown Journal on Poverty Law and Policy*, 17:165–220.

Johnson, J. G., Cohen, P., Kasen, S., and Brook, J. J. (2002). Childhood adversities associated with risk for eating disorders or weight problems during adolescence or early adulthood. *American Journal of Psychiatry*, 159, no. 3: 394–400.

Johnson, P. (2005). Obesity: Epidemic or myth? *Committee for Skeptical Inquiry*, 29, no. 5 (October).

Johnson, R., Panely, C., and Wang, M. (2001). Associations between the milk mothers drink and the milk consumed by their school-aged children. *Family Economics and Nutrition Review*, 13, no. 1: 27–36.

Jones, A., and Panter, J. (2010). Availability and accessibility in physical activity environments. In A. A. Lake, T. G. Townshend, and S. Alvanides (Eds.), *Obesogenic environments: Complexities, perceptions, and objective measures* (pp. 41–61). Oxford, UK: Blackwell Publishing.

Jones, J., and Barry, M. M. (2011). Exploring the relationship between synergy and partnership functioning factors in health promotion partnerships. *Health Promotion International*, 29, no. 6: 683–698.

Joshi, A., Azuma, A. M., and Feenstra, G. (2008). Do farm-to-school programs make a difference? Findings and future research needs. *Journal of Hunger and Environmental Nutrition*, 3, no. 2/3: 229–246.

Kaiser, M. L. (2011). Food security: An ecological-social analysis to promote social development. *Journal of Community Practice*, 19, no. 1: 62–79.

Kanagui-Munoz, M., Garriott, P. O., Flores, L. Y., Cho, S., and Groves, J. (2011). Latina/o food industry employees' work experiences: Work behaviors, facilitators, motivators, training preferences, and perceptions. *Journal of Career Development*, 39, no. 1: 118–139.

Kant, A., and Graubard, B. (2007). Secular trends in the association of socioeconomic position with self-reported dietary attributes and biomarkers in the US population: National Health and Nutrition Examination Survey (NHANES) 1971–1975 to NHANES 1999–2002. *Public Health Nutrition*, 10, no. 2: 158–167.

Kasser, T. (2009). Psychological need satisfaction, personal well-being, and ecological sustainability. *Ecopsychology*, 1, no. 4: 175–180.

Kaufman, L., and Karpati, A. (2007). Understanding the sociocultural roots of childhood obesity: Food practices among Latino families of Bushwick, Brooklyn. *Social Science and Medicine*, 64, no. 11: 2177–2188.

Kaushal, N. (2009). Adversities of acculturation? Prevalence of obesity among immigrants. *Health Economics*, 18, no. 4: 291–303.

Kegler, M. C., Norton, B. L., and Aronson, R. (2007). Skill improvement among coalition members in the California Healthy Cities and Communities Program. *Health Education Research*, 22, no. 3: 450–457.

Kegler, M. C., Oman, R. F., Vesely, S. K., McLeroy, K. R., Aspy, C. B., Rodine, S., and Marshall, L. (2005). Relationships among youth assets and neighborhood and community resources. *Health Education and Behavior*, 32, no. 3: 380–397.

Kegler, M. C., Rigler, J., and Honeycutt, S. (2010). How does community context influence coalition in the formation stage? A multiple case study based on the Community Coalition Action Theory. *BMC Public Health*, 10, no. 1: 90.

Kegler, M. C., Rigler, J., and Honeycutt, S. (2011). The role of community context in planning and implementing community-based health promotion projects. *Evaluation and Program Planning*, 34, no. 3: 246–253.

Kelley, M. A., Benson, M., Estrella, M., and Lugardo, J. (2009). *Jovenes sin fronteras: Latino youth take action for social justice and well-being.* Chicago: University of Illinois at Chicago, Great Cities Institute.

Kersh, R., and Morone, J. (2002). The politics of obesity: Seven steps to government action. *Health Affairs*, 21, no. 6: 142–153.

Khan, L. K., Sobush, K., Keener, D., Goodman, K., Lowry, A., Kakietek, J., and Zaro, S. (2009). Recommended community strategies and measurements to prevent obesity in the United States. *Morbidity and Mortality Weekly Report*, 58 (RR07): 1–26.

Kim, D. (2008). Blues from the neighborhood? Neighborhood characteristics and depression. *Epidemiologic Reviews*, 30, no. 1: 101–117.

Kim, S., Flaskerud, J. H., Koniak-Griffin, D., and Dixon, E. (2005). Using community-partnered participatory research to address health disparities in Latino communities. *Journal of the Association of Nurses in AIDS Care*, 21, no. 4: 199–209.

Kimbro, R. T., Brooks-Gunn, J., and McLanahan, S. (2007). Racial and ethnic differentials in overweight and obesity among 3-year-old children. *American Journal of Public Health*, 97, no. 2: 298–305.

King, C., and Siegel, M. (2001, August 16). The Master Settlement Agreement with the tobacco industry and cigarette advertising in magazines. *New England Journal of Medicine*, 345, no. 7: 505–511.

King, D. W., Vigil, I. T., Herrera, A. P., Hajek, R. A., and Jones, L. A. (2007). Working toward social justice: Center on Research on Minority Health Summer

Workshop on Hispanic Disparities. *California Journal of Health Promotion*, 5, special issue: 1–8.

King, L., Gill, T., Allender, S., and Swinburn, B. (2011). Best practice principles for community-based obesity prevention: Development, content, and application. *Obesity Reviews*, 12, no. 5: 329–338.

Kipke, M. D., Iverson, E., Moore, D., Booker, C., Ruelas, V., Peters, A. L., and Kaufman, F. (2007). Food and park environments: Neighborhood-level risks for childhood obesity in East Los Angeles. *Journal of Adolescent Health*, 40, no. 4: 325–333.

Kirshner, B. (2008). Guided participation in three youth action organizations: Facilitation, apprenticeship, and joint work. *Journal of the Learning Sciences*, 17, no. 1: 60–101.

Kirshner, B. (2009). "Power in numbers": Youth organizing as a context for exploring civic identity. *Journal of Research on Adolescence*, 19, no. 3: 414–440.

Kirshner, B., and Geil, K. (2010). "I'm about to really bring it!" Access points between youth activists and adult community leaders. *Children, Youth, and Environment*, 20, no. 1: 1–37.

Klein, J. D., and Dietz, W. (2010). Childhood obesity: The new tobacco. *Health Affairs*, 29, no. 3: 388–392.

Klein, R. (2006). Review of *The obesity epidemic: Science and ideology*. *International Journal of Epidemiology*, 351, no. 3: 207–208.

Kolata, G. (2011, October 27). Study shows why it's hard to keep weight off. *New York Times*, p. A14.

Kolotkin, R. L., Binks, M., Crosby, R. D., Ostebye, T., Gress, R. E., and Adams, T. D. (2006). Obesity and sexual quality of life. *Obesity*, 14, no. 3: 472–479.

Koplan, J. P., Liverman, C. T., and Kraak, V. I. (2005). *Preventing childhood obesity: Health in the balance*. Washington, DC: National Academies Press.

Kown, S. A. (2008). Moving from complaints to action: Oppositional consciousness and collective action in a political community. *Anthropology and Education Quarterly*, 39, no. 1: 59–76.

Krebs, N. F., Himes, J. H., Jacobson, D., Nicklas, T. A., Guilday, P., and Styne, D. (2007). Assessment of child and adolescent overweight and obesity. *Pediatrics*, 120, suppl.: S193–S228.

Krenichi, R. (2006). 'The only place to go and be in the city': Women talk about exercise, being outdoors, and the meanings of a large urban park. *Health and Place*, 12, no. 4: 631–643.

Krukowski, R. A., Lueders, N. K., Prewitt, T. E., Williams, D. K., and Smith, D. (2010). Obesity treatment tailored for a Catholic faith community: A feasibility study. *Journal of Health Psychology*, 15, no. 3: 382–390.

Kuczmarski, R. J. (2007). What is obesity? Definitions matter. In S. Kumanyika and R. C. Brownson (Eds.), *Handbook of obesity prevention: A resource for health professionals* (pp. 25–11). New York: Springer

Kuczmarski, R. J., Flegal, K. M., Campbell, S. M., and Johnson, C. L. (1994). Increasing prevalence of overweight among U.S. adults. The National Health and Nutrition Examination Surveys, 1960–1991. *Journal of the American Medical Association*, 272, 205–211.

Kumanyika, S. K. (2001). Obesity treatment in minorities. In T. A. Wadden and A. J. Stunkard (Eds.), *Handbook of obesity treatment* (pp. 416–446). New York: Guilford Press.

Kumanyika, S. K. (2005). Obesity, health disparities, and prevention paradigms: Hard questions and hard choices. *Preventing Chronic Disorders*, 2, no. 4: A02, Epub 2005.

Kumanyika, S. K. (2007). Obesity prevention concepts and frameworks. In S. Kumanyika and R. C. Brownson (Eds.), *Handbook of obesity prevention: A resource for health professionals* (pp. 85–114). New York: Springer.

Kumanyika, S. K. (2008a). Environmental influences on childhood obesity: Ethnic and cultural influences in context. *Physiology and Behavior*, 94, no. 1: 61–70.

Kumanyika, S. K. (2008b). Ethnic minorities and weight control research priorities: Where are we now and where do we need to be? *Preventive Medicine*, 47, no. 6: 583–586.

Kumanyika, S. K., and Brownson, R. C. (Eds.). (2007). *Handbook of obesity prevention: A resource for health professionals*. New York: Springer.

Kumanyika, S. K., Obarzanek, E., Stettler, N., Bell, R., Field, A. E., Fortmann, S. P., Franklin, B. A., Gillman, M. W., Lewis, C. E., Poston II, W. C., Stevens, J., and Hong, Y. (2008). Population-based prevention of obesity. *Circulation*, 118: 428–464.

Kwan, S. (2008). Framing the fat body: Contested meanings between government, activists, and industry. *Sociological Inquiry*, 79, no. 1: 25–50.

Kwate, N. O. A., Yau, C.-Y., Loh, J.-M., and Williams, D. (2008). Fried chicken and fresh apples: Racial segregation as a fundamental cause of fast food density in black neighborhoods. *Health and Place*, 14, no. 1: 32–41.

L.A. Health. (2003). *Obesity on the rise*. Los Angeles: County of Los Angeles Department of Health Services.

L.A. Health Trends. (2006). *The obesity epidemic in Los Angeles County adults*. Los Angeles: County of Los Angeles Department of Health Services.

Lacey, T. A., and Wright, B. (2009, November). Occupational employment projections to 2018. *Monthly Labor Review*, 82–123.

Lake, A., and Midgley, J. L. (2010). Food policy and food governance—changing behaviours. In A. A. Lake, T. G. Townshend, and S. Alvanides (Eds.), *Obesogenic environments: Complexities, perceptions, and objective measures* (pp. 165–182). Oxford, UK: Blackwell Publishing.

Lake, A., and Townshend, T. (2006). Obesogenic environments: Exploring the built and food environments. *Perspectives in Public Health*, 126, no. 6: 262–267.

Lake, A. A., Townshend, T. G., and Alvanides, S. (Eds.). (2010). *Obesogenic environments: Complexities, perceptions, and objective measures.* Oxford, UK: Blackwell Publishing.

Landigan, P. J., Rauh, V. A., and Galvez, M. P. (2010). Environmental justice and the health of children. *Mount Sinai Journal of Medicine: A Journal of Translational and Personalized Medicine,* 77, no. 2: 178–187.

Landry, S. M., and Chakraborty, J. (2009). Street trees and equity: The spatial distribution of an urban amenity. *Environment and Planning,* 41, no. 10: 2651–2670.

Lantz, P. M., Lichtenstein, R. L., and Pollack, H. A. (2007). Health policy approaches to population health: The limits of medicalization. *Health Affairs,* 26, no. 5: 1253–1257.

Laqueur, T., (1999). *Making sex: Body and gender from the Greeks to Freud.* Cambridge, MA: Harvard University Press.

Lara, M., Gamboa, C., Kahramanian, M. I., Morales, L. S., and Bautista, D. E. (2005). Acculturation and Latino health in the United States: A review of the literature and its sociopolitical context. *Annual Review of Public Health,* 26:367–397.

Larsen, K., and Gilliland, J. (2009). A farmers' market in a food desert: Evaluating impacts on the price and availability of healthy food. *Health and Place,* 15, no. 4: 1158–1162.

Larson, N. K. (2005). *Tending nature's classroom: A qualitative examination of motivations and values of educational place-making at Troy Gardens.* Madison: University of Wisconsin.

Larson, N., and Story, M. (2009). A review of environmental influences on food choices. *Annals of Behavioral Medicine,* 38, suppl. 1: S56–S73.

Latino Coalition for a Healthy California. (2006). *Obesity in Latino communities.* Sacramento: Author.

Latino Health Access. (2009, October 16). *Community health crusade.* Santa Ana, CA: Author.

Lautenschlager, L., and Smith, C. (2007). Understanding gardening and dietary habits among youth garden program participants using the theory of planned behavior. *Appetite,* 49, no. 1: 122–130.

Lavelle, M. (Ed.). (1994). *"Information please"Environmental Almanac. World Resource Institute.* Boston: Houghton-Mifflin.

Lawrence, J. M., et al. (2009). Diabetes in Hispanic American youth: Prevalence, incidence, demographics, and clinical characteristics: The SEARCH for Diabetes in Youth Study. *Diabetes Care,* 32, suppl. 2: S123–S132.

Lawrence, R. G. (2004). Framing obesity: The evolution of news discourse on a public health issue. *Harvard International Journal of Press/Politics,* 9, no. 3: 56–75.

Lawson, L. J. (2005). *City bountiful: A century of community gardening in America.* Berkeley: University of California Press.

Lazar, K. (2011, March 7). Shortage of grocers plagues Mass. cities. *Boston Globe,* pp. A1, A10.

Lee, C. (2002). Environmental justice: Building a unified vision of health and the environment. *Environmental Health Perspectives*, 110, no. 2: 141–144.

Lee, J. M., Lim, S., Zoellner, J., Burt, B. A., Sandretto, M., Sohn, W., and Ismail, A. I. (2010). Don't children grow out of their obesity? Weight transitions in early childhood. *Clinical Pediatrics*, 49, no. 5: 466–469.

Lee, R. E., and Cubbin, C. (2009). Striding toward social justice: The ecologic milieu of physical activity. *Exercise and Sport Science Review*, 37, no. 1: 10–17.

Lester, J. P., Allen, D. W., and Hill, K. M. (2001). *Environmental injustice in the United States: Myths and realities*. Boulder, CO: Westview Press.

Levenstein, H. A. (1993). *Paradox of plenty: A social history of eating in modern America*. New York: Oxford University Press.

Levenstein, H. A. (2003). *Revolution at the table: The transformation of the American diet*. Berkeley: University of California Press.

Levernance, R. R., Williams, R. L., Sussman, A., and Crabtree, B. F. (2007). Obesity counseling and guidelines in primary care. *American Journal of Preventive Medicine*, 32, no. 4: 334–339.

Levi, J., Vinter, S., Richardson, L., St. Laurent, R., and Segal, L. M. (2009). *F as in fat: How obesity policies are failing in America*. Washington, DC: Trust for America's Health.

Levi, J., Vinter, S., St. Laurent, R., and Segal, L. M. (2010). *F as in fat: How obesity threatens America's future*. Washington, DC: Trust for America's Health.

Levine, M. A. (2012). Preface. In M. A. Levine (Ed.), *Urban society annual edition* (pp. iv–vi). New York: McGraw-Hill.

Levkoe, C. Z. (2006). Learning democracy through food justice movements. *Agriculture and Human Values*, 23, no. 1: 89–98.

Lewis, L. B., Galloway-Gillian, L., Flynn, G., Nomachu, J., Keener, L. C., and Sloane, D. C. (2011). Transforming the urban food desert from the grassroots up: A model for community change. *Family and Community Health*, 11, suppl.: S92–S101.

Lewis-Charp, H., Yu, H. C., and Soukamneuth, S. (2005). Civic activist approaches for engaging youth in social justice. In S. Ginwright, P. Noguera, and J. Cammarota (Eds.), *Beyond resistance: Youth activism and community change* (pp. 21–57). New York: Routledge.

Liburd, L. C. (Ed.). (2010a). *Diabetes and health disparities: Community-based approaches for racial and ethnic populations*. New York: Springer.

Liburd, L. C. (2010b). The co-emergence of the diabetes and obesity epidemics in racial and ethnic populations. In L. C. Liburd (Ed.), *Diabetes and health disparities: Community-based approaches for racial and ethnic populations* (pp. 61–84). New York: Springer.

Liburd, L. C. (2010c). Culture, meaning, and obesity among college-educated African-American women: An anthropological perspective. In L. C. Liburd (Ed.), *Diabetes and health disparities: Community-based approaches for racial and ethnic populations* (pp. 85–117). New York: Springer.

Lindley, P. A., Bhaduri, A., Sharma, D. S., and Govindji, R. (2011). Strengthening underprivileged communities: Strengths-based approaches as a force for positive social change in communities. In R. Biswas-Diena (Ed.), *Positive psychology as social change* (pp. 141–156). New York: Springer.

Liou, D., and Bauer, K. (2010). Obesity perceptions among Chinese Americans: The interface of traditional Chinese and American values. *Food, Culture, and Society: An International Journal of Multidisciplinary Research*, 13, no. 3: 351–369.

Lipinski, J. (2010, September 19). A commune grows in Brooklyn: Bushwick embraces the collective way of life. *New York Times* (Sunday Styles), pp. 1, 8.

Lissner, L. (2002). Measuring food intake in studies of obesity. *Public Health Nutrition*, 5, no. 6A: 889–892.

Liu, J., Probst, J. C., Harun, N., Bennett, K. J., and Torres, M. E. (2009). Acculturation, physical activity, and obesity among Hispanic adolescents. *Ethnicity and Health*, 14, no. 5: 509–525.

Livingston, M. (2008) Alcohol outlet density and assault: A spatial analysis. *Addiction*, 103, no. 4: 619–628.

Lobstein, T., Baur, L., and Uauy, R. (2004). Obesity in children and young adults: A crisis in public health. *Obesity Reviews*, 5, suppl. 1: 4–85.

Lopez, R. (2004). Urban sprawl and risk for being overweight or obese. *American Journal of Public Health*, 94, no. 9: 1574–1579.

Lopez, R., Campbell, R., and Jennings, J. (2008). The Boston Schoolyard initiative: A public-private partnership for rebuilding urban play spaces. *Journal of Health Politics, Policy, and Law*, 33, no. 3: 617–638.

Lopez, R. P., and Hynes, H. P. (2006). Obesity, physical activity, and the urban environment: Public health research needs. *Environmental Health: A Global Access Science Source* 5, no. 1: 1–16.

Lorenc, T., Harden, A., Brunton, G., and Oakley, A. (2008). *Including diverse groups of children and young people in health promotion and public health research: A review of methodology and practice*. London: EPPI-Centre, Social Service Research Unit, University of London.

Loukaiton-Sideris, A. (2006). Is it safe to walk? Neighborhood safety and security considerations and their effects on walking. *Journal of Planning Literature*, 20, no. 3: 219–232.

Lovasi, G. S., Hutson, M. A., Guerra, M., and Neckerman, K. M. (2010). Built environments and obesity in disadvantaged populations. *Epidemiologic Reviews*, 31, no. 1: 7–20.

Lowrie, K. W., Solitare, L., and Himmelfarb, K. (2011). Building capacity for community-based brownfields remediation and redevelopment: An innovative technical assistance model. *Remediation: The Journal of Environmental Cleanup Costs, Technologies, and Techniques*, 21, no. 2: 101–115.

Ludwig, D. S. (2007). Childhood obesity—The shape of things to come. *New England Journal of Medicine*, 357, no. 23: 2325–2327.

Ludwig, D. S., and Nestle, M. (2008). Can the food industry play a constructive role in the obesity epidemic? *Journal of the American Medical Association*, 300, no. 5: 1808–1811.

Ludwig, D. S., and Pollack, H. A. (2009). Obesity and the economy: From crisis to opportunity. *Journal of the American Medical Association*, 301, no. 5: 533–535.

Lumeng, J. C., Appugliese, D., Cabral, H. J., Bradley, R. H., and Zuckerman, B. (2006). Neighborhood safety and overweight status in children. *Archives of Pediatrics*, 160, no. 1: 25–31.

Lund, D. E. (2010). *Drawing insights from former youth leaders in social justice activism*. Calgary, Canada: University of Calgary.

Lund, D. E., and Nabavi, M. (2008). Understanding student anti-racism activism to foster social justice in schools. *International Journal of Multicultural Education*, 10, no. 1: 1–20.

Lutz, A. E., Swisher, M. E., and Brennan, M. A. (2010). *Defining community food security*. Gainesville: University of Florida.

Lyson, T. A. (2004). *Civic agriculture: Reconnecting farm, food, and community*. Medford, MA: Tufts University Press.

Lyson, T. A., Gillespie, G. W., and Hilchey, D. (1995). Farmers' markets and the local community: Bridging the formal and informal economy. *American Journal of Alternative Agriculture*, 10, no. 1: 108–113.

Macdonald, E. (2007). Wasted space/potential place: Reconsidering urban streets. *Places*, 19, no. 1: 22–27.

Macintyre, S., Ellaway, A., and Cummins, S. (2002). Place effects on health: How can we conceptualise, operationalise and measure them? *Social Science and Medicine*, 55, no. 1: 125–139.

Mackett, R. L. (2010). Active travel. In A. A. Lake, T. G. Townshend, and S. Alvanides (Eds.), *Obesogenic environments: Complexities, perceptions, and objective measures* (pp. 117–131). Oxford, UK: Blackwell Publishing.

Main, E. (2010, September 10). *Dumpster-dining: Should you try it?* Rodale Institute. http:www.rodale.com/food-industry-waste?page-0%2C1). Accessed 9/10/10.

Mair, H., Sumna, J., and Rotteau, L. (2008). The politics of eating: Food practices as critically reflexive leisure. *Leisure/Loisir*, 32, no. 2: 379–405.

Maloni, M. J., and Brown, M. E. (2006). Corporate social responsibility in the supply chain: An application in the food industry. *Journal of Business Ethics*, 68, no. 1: 35–52.

Malterud, K., and Tonstad, S. (2009). Preventing obesity: Challenges and pitfalls for health promotion. *Patient Education and Counseling*, 76, no. 2: 254–259.

Mangurian, C., Stowe, M., and Devlin, M. J. (2009). Obesity treatment for urban, low-income Latinos with severe mental illness. *Psychiatric Services*, 60, no. 8: 1139.

Mantel, B. (2010). Preventing obesity: Do Americans face too many obstacles to healthy eating? *Congressional Quarterly Researcher*, 20, no. 34: 1–36.

Marcias, T. (2008). Working toward a just, equitable, and local food system: The social impact of community-based agriculture. *Social Science Quarterly*, 89, no. 5: 1086–1101.

Margellos-Anast, H., Shah, A. M., and Whitman, S. (2008). Prevalence of obesity among children in six Chicago communities: Findings from a health survey. *Public Health Reports*, 123, no. 1: 117–123.

Marmot, M., and Wilkinson, R. G. (2006). *Social determinants of health*. New York: Oxford University Press.

Marshall, J. D., Brauer, M., and Frank, L. D. (2009). Healthy neighborhoods: Walkability and air pollution. *Environmental Health Perspectives*, 117, no. 11: 1752–1759.

Marshall, P. (2004). Advertising overload: Are more restrictions needed? *Congressional Quarterly Researcher*, 11, no. 3: 1–33.

Martin, A. (2009, March 21). Is a food revolution now in session? *New York Times*, p. A21.

Martin, K. S., and Ferris, A. M. (2007). Food insecurity and gender are risk factors for obesity. *Journal of Nutrition Education and Behavior*, 39, no. 1: 31–36.

Mascie-Taylor, C. G. N., and Goto, R. (2007). Human variation and body mass index: A review of the universality of BMI cut-offs, gender and urban-rural differences, and secular changes. *Journal of Physiological Anthropology*, 26, no. 2: 109–112.

Mason, A. R., Hill, R. C., Myers, L. A., and Street, A. D. (2008). Establishing the economics of engaging communities in health promotion: What is desirable, what is feasible. *Critical Public Health*, 18, no. 3: 285–297.

Masuda, J. R., Poland, B., and Baxter, J. (2010). Reaching for environmental health justice: Canadian experiences for a comprehensive research, policy, and advocacy agenda in health promotion. *Health Promotion International*. doi:10.1093/heapro/daq041. Accessed 8/6/10.

Maximova, K., McGrath, J. J., Barnett, T., O' Loughlin, J., Paradis, G., and Lambert, M. (2008). Do you see what I see? Weight status misperceptions and exposure to obesity among children and adolescents. *International Journal of Obesity*, 32, no. 6: 1008–1015.

Maxwell, B., and Jacobson, M. (1989). *Marketing disease to Hispanics*. Washington, DC: Center for Science in the Public Interest.

Mayer, K. (2009). Childhood obesity prevention: Focusing on the community food environment. *Family and Community Health*, 32, no. 3: 257–270.

McAleese, J. D., and Rankin, L. L. (2007). Garden-based nutrition education affects fruit and vegetable consumption in sixth-grade adolescents. *Journal of the American Dietetic Association*, 107, no. 4: 662–665.

McAlexander, K. M., Banda, J. A., McAlexander, J. W., and Lee, R. E. (2009). Physical activity resource attributes and obesity in low-income African Americans. *Journal of Urban Health*, 86, no. 5: 696–707.

McClintock, N. (2008). *From industrial garden to food desert: Unearthing the root structure of urban agriculture in Oakland, California*. Berkeley: University of California, Institute for the Study of Social Change.

McCormack, L. A., Laska, M. N., Larson, N. I., and Story, M. (2010). Review of the nutritional implications of farmers' markets and community gardens: A call for evaluation and research efforts. *Journal of the American Dietetic Association*, 110, no. 3: 399–408.

McCormick, B. (2007). Economic costs of obesity and the case for government intervention. *Obesity Reviews*, 8, suppl. 1: 161–164.

McCullum, C., Desjardins, E., Kraak, V. I., Ladipo, P., and Costello, H. (2005). Evidence-based strategies to build community food security. *Journal of American Dietetic Association*, 105, no. 2: 278–283.

Mcintyre, S., Macdonald, L., and Ellaway, A. (2008). A lack of agreement between measured and self-reported distance from public green parks in Glasgow, Scotland. *International Journal of Behavioral Nutrition and Physical Activity*, 5, no. 1: 26.

McKinnon, R. A. (2010). A rationale for policy intervention in reducing obesity. *Virtual Mentor*, 12, no. 4: 309–315.

McLaren, L. (2007). Socioeconomic status and obesity. *Epidemiologic Reviews*, 29, no. 1: 29–48.

McLean, L. (2007). Socioeconomic status and obesity. *Epidemiologic Reviews*, 29, no. 1: 29–48.

McLean, L., Edwards, N., Garrard, M., Sims-Jones, N., Clinton, K., and Ashley, L. (2009). Obesity, stigma, and public health planning. *Health Promotion International*, 24, no. 1: 88–93.

McMillan, T. (2008, May 7). Urban farmers' crops go from vacant lot to market. *New York Times*, p. A17.

McQueen, D., and Jones, C. (Eds.). (2007). *Global perspectives on health promotion effectiveness*. New York: Springer.

MedicAnimal.com. (2010, November 26). Insurer reveals extent of canine obesity. Author.

Medina, J. (2011, January 16). In South Los Angeles, new fast-food spots get a "no, thanks." *New York Times*, p. 15.

Mediratta, R. (2006). A rising movement. *National Civic Review*, 126, Spring: 15–22.

Mehta, N. K., and Chang, V. W. (2008). Weight status and restaurant availability: A multilevel analysis. *American Journal of Preventive Medicine*, 34, no. 2: 127–133.

Mehta, V. (2007). Lively streets: Determining environmental characteristics to support social behaviors. *Journal of Planning Education and Research*, 27, no. 2: 165–187.

Meislik, A. (2004). Weighing in on the scale of justice: The obesity epidemic and litigations against the food industry. *Arizona Law Review*, 46: 781–814.

Mercier, J. (2009). Equity, social justice, and sustainable urban transportation in the twenty-first century. *Administrative Theory and Praxis*, 31, no. 2: 145–163.

Merzel, C., and D'Afflitti, J. (2003). Reconsidering community-based health promotion: Promise, performance, and potential. *American Journal of Public Health*, 93, no. 4: 557–574.

Meyer, K. (2008). Prevention of obesity and physical inactivity—a socio-cultural challenge. *Journal of Public Health*, 16, no. 1: 1–2.

Michael, Y. L., and Yen, I. H. (2009). Invited commentary: Built environment and obesity among older adults—can neighborhood-level policy interventions make a difference? *American Journal of Epidemiology*, 169, no. 4: 409–412.

Mikkelsen, L., Erikson, C. S., Sims, J., and Nestle, M. (2010). Creating healthy food environments to prevent chronic diseases. In L. Cohen, V. Chavez, and S. Chehimi (Eds.), *Prevention is primary: Strategies for community well-being* (pp. 291–322). San Francisco: Jossey-Bass.

Miner, C. (2010). Taking root in the city: Urban agriculture is changing our relationship with food—for good. *Ode: For Intelligent Optimists*, July/August, 40–43.

Minihan, P. M., Fitch, S. N., and Must, A. (2007). What does the epidemic of childhood obesity mean for children with special health care needs? *Journal of Law, Medicine, and Ethics*, 35, no. 1: 61–77.

Minkler, M., and Wallerstein, N. (Eds.). (2003). *Community-based participatory research for health*. San Francisco: Jossey-Bass.

Mirza, H. M., Davis, D., and Yanovski, A. (2005). Body dissatisfaction, self-esteem, and overweight among inner-city Hispanic children and adolescents. *Journal of Adolescent Health*, 36, no. 3: e16–267–e20.

Mitchell, D. (2003). *The right to the city: Social justice and the fight for public space*. New York: Guilford Press.

Mittelmark, M. B. (2008). Editorial. Health promotion: A professional community for social justice. *Promotion and Education*, 15, no. 2: 3–5.

Miyake, K. K., Maroko, A. R., Grady, K. L., Maantay, J. A., and Arno, P. S. (2010). Not just a walk in the park: Methodological improvements for determining environmental justice Implications of park access in New York City for the promotion of physical activity. *Cities and the Environment*, 3, no. 1: 1–17.

MkNelly, B. (2009). *Food Stamp Program and obesity: Brief summary of research*. Sacramento: California Department of Public Health, Public Health Institute.

Mobach, P., and Catlow, L. (2007). *CHAMPS—Children's Healthy Activities Mentoring Program for Schools*. Paper presented at the 9th National Rural Health Conference, Albury, NSW.

Mohai, P., and Saha, R. (2006). Reassessing racial and socioeconomic disparities in environmental justice research. *Demography*, 43, no. 2: 383–399.

Mohn, T. (2010, October 19). Fresh from the roof: Hotels take "locally grown" the logical next step. *New York Times*, p. B7.

Moloni, M. J., and Brown, M. E. (2006). Corporate social responsibilities in the supply chain: An application in the food industry. *Journal of Business Ethics*, 68, no. 1: 35–52.

Monaghan, L. F., Hollands, R., and Pritchard, G. (2010). Obesity epidemic entrepreneurs· Types, practices, and interests. *Body and Society*, 16, no. 2: 37–71.

Moniz, C. (2010). Social work and the social determinants of health perspective: A good fit. *Health and Social Work*, 35, no. 4: 310–313.

Moore, J. B., Jillcott, S. B., Shores, K. A., Evenson, K. R., Brownson, R. C., and Novick, L. F. (2010). A qualitative examination of perceived barriers and facilitators of physical activity for urban and rural youth. *Health Education Research*, 25, no. 2: 355–367.

Morbidity and Mortality Weekly Report. (2009). Obesity prevalence among low-income, preschool-aged children—United States, 1998–2008, 303, no. 1: 769–773.

Morgan, A., and Ziglio, E. (2007). Revitalizing the evidence base for public health: An assets model. *Promotion and Education*, 14, suppl. 2: 17–22.

Morgan, K. (2009). Feeding the city: The challenge of urban food planning. *International Planning Studies*, 14, no. 4: 341–348.

Morgan, K. (2010). Local and green, global and fair: The ethical foodscape and the politics of care. *Environment and Planning*, 42, no. 12: 1852–1867.

Morland, K., Diez Roux, A. V., and Wing, S. (2006). Supermarkets, other food stores, and obesity: The atherosclerosis risk in communities study. *American Journal of Preventive Medicine*, 30, no. 4: 333–339.

Morland, K., and Everson, K. R. (2009). Obesity prevalence and the local food environment. *Health and Place*, 15, no. 2: 491–495.

Morland, K., and Filomena, S. (2008). The utilization of local food environments by urban seniors. *Preventive Medicine*, 47, no. 3: 289–293.

Morland, K., and Wing, S. (2007). Food justice and health in communities of color. In R. D. Bullard (Ed.), *Growing smarter: Achieving livable communities, environmental justice, and regional equity* (pp. 171–188). Cambridge, MA: MIT Press.

Moss, M. (2011). Philadelphia school battles students' bad eating habits, on campus and off. *New York Times*, pp. A14, A16.

Mougeot, L. J. A. (1993). Overview—urban food self-reliance: Significance and prospects. *International Development Research Centre*, 21, no. 3: 1–3.

MSNBC.com. (2011). Illegal worker crackdown bites Chipotle. http://www.msnbc .com/id/41469433/ns/business-consumer_news/. Accessed 4/11/11.

Muennig, P., Lubetkin, E., Jia, H., and Franks, P. (2006). Gender and the burden of disease attributable to obesity. *American Journal of Public Health*, 96, no. 9: 1662–1668.

Mundy, A. (2002). *Dispensing with the truth: The victims, the drug companies, and the dramatic story behind the battle over Fen-Phen*. New York: St. Martin's Press.

Munger, L. T. (2003–2004). Comment: Is Ronald McDonald the next Joe Camel? Regulating fast food advertisements targeting children in light of the American overweight and obesity epidemic. *Connecticut Public Interest Law Journal*, 3, no. 2: 456–480.

Murrock, C. J., and Gary, F. A. (2010). Culturally specific dance to reduce obesity in African American women. *Health Promotion Practice*, 11, no. 4: 465–473.

Mustafa, K., MacRae, R., and Mougeot, L. J. A. (Eds.). (1999). *For hunger-proof cities: Sustainable urban food systems.* Ottawa, Canada: International Development Research Centre.

Nafiu, O. O., Burke, C., Lee, J., Vaepel-Lewis, T., Malviya, S., and Tremper, K. K. (2010). Neck circumference as a screening measure for identifying children with high body mass index. *Pediatrics*, 126, no. 2: e306–e310.

Nanney, M. S. (2007). Obesity prevention during preschool and elementary school-age years. In S. Kumanyika and R. C. Brownson (Eds.), *Handbook of obesity prevention: A resource for health professionals* (pp. 429–458). New York: Springer.

National Association of Social Workers. (2008). *Code of ethics.* Washington, DC: Author.

Nault, K., Fitzpatrick, M., and Howard, P. H. (2010). Engaging youth in food environments research: The role of participation. *Journal of Hunger and Environmental Nutrition*, 5, no. 2: 174–190.

Neergaard, L. (2010, September 21). Cost of obesity? Over $4,000 if you're a woman. msnbc.com. http://www.msnbc.msn.com/id/39276141/ns/health-diet_and_nutrition/. Accessed 9/21/10.

Neovius, K., Johannson, K., Kark, M., and Neovius, M. (2009). Obesity status and sick leave: A systematic review. *Obesity Reviews*, 10, no. 1: 17–27.

Neovius, M., Janson, A., and Rossner, S. (2006). Prevalence of obesity in Sweden. *Obesity Reviews*, 7, no. 1: 1–3.

Nestle, M. (2007). *Food politics: How the food industry influences nutrition and health.* Berkeley: University of California Press.

Neuman, W. (2011, April 29). U.S. seeks stricter limits on food advertising aimed at children. *New York Times*, pp. A1, B4.

Neumark-Szainer, D., Haines, J., Robinson-O'Brien, R., Hannan, P. J., Robins, M., Morris, B., and Petrich, C. A. (2008). "Ready. Set. ACTION!" A theater-based obesity prevention program for children: A feasibility study. *Health Education Research*, 24, no. 3: 407–420.

Nevill, A. M., Stewart, A. D., Olds, T., and Holder, R. (2006). Relationship between adiposity and body size reveals limitations of BMI. *American Journal of Physical Anthropology*, 129, no. 2: 151–156.

New Economics. (2010). *Food and social justice.* London: Author.

Newman, A. M. (2009). Obesity in older adults. *Online Journal of Issues in Nursing*, 14, no. 1.

Nicheles, J. (2006). *Developing a social marketing initiative to prevent obesity and promote healthy lifestyle behaviors in Chicago families.* Paper presented at the American Public Health Association annual meeting, Boston, MA.

Noguera, P., and Cannella, C. M. (2006). Youth agency, resistance, and civic activism: The public commitment to social justice. In S. Ginwright, P. Noguera, and J. Cammarota (Eds.), *Beyond resistance: Youth activism and community change* (pp. 333–347). New York: Routledge.

Nordahl, D. (2009). *Public produce: The new urban agriculture.* Washington, DC: Island Press.

Odoms-Young, A. M., Zenk, S., and Mason, M. (2009). Measuring food availability and access in African-American communities: Implications for interventions and policy. *American Journal of Preventive Medicine,* 36, suppl. 4: S145–S150.

Office of Minority Health. (2007). *HHS fact sheet: Minority health disparities at a glance.* Washington, DC: Author.

Office of Minority Health. (2010a). *Diabetes and Asian and Pacific Islanders.* Washington, DC: Author.

Office of Minority Health. (2010b). *Diabetes and Hispanic Americans.* Washington, DC: Author.

Office of Minority Health. (2010c). *Diabetes and Native Hawaiians/Pacific Islanders.* Washington, DC: Author.

Office of Minority Health. (2010d). *Statistics on African-Americans and strokes.* Washington, DC: Author.

Office of Minority Health. (2010e). *Statistics on American Indians/Alaska Natives and strokes.* Washington, DC: Author.

Office of Minority Health. (2010f). *Statistics on Asian-Americans and strokes.* Washington, DC: Author.

Office of Minority Health. (2010g). *Statistics on Hispanic-Americans and strokes.* Washington, D.C: Author.

Office of Minority Health. (2010h). *Statistics on Native Hawaiians/Pacific Islanders and strokes.* Washington, DC: Author.

Office of Minority Health. (2011a). *Obesity and African-Americans.* Washington, DC: Author.

Office of Minority Health. (2011b). *Obesity and American Indians/Alaska Natives.* Washington, DC: Author.

Office of Minority Health. (2011c). *Obesity and Hispanics.* Washington, DC: Author.

Office of Minority Health. (2011d). *Obesity and Native Hawaiians/Pacific Islanders.* Washington, DC: Author.

Office of Minority Health. (2011e). *Obesity and Asian-Americans.* Washington, DC: Author.

Ogden, C. L., Carroll, M. D., Curtin, L. R., McDowell, M. A., Tabak, C. J., and Flegal, K. M. (2006). Prevalence of overweight and obesity in the United States, 1999–2004. *Journal of the American Medical Association,* 295, no. 13: 1549–1555.

Ogden, C. L., Yanovski, S. Z., Carroll, M. D., and Flegal, K. M. (2007). The epidemiology of obesity. *Gastroenterology,* 132, no. 2: 2087–2102.

Olden, K., Ramos, R. M., and Freudenberg, N. (2009). To reduce urban disparities in health, strengthen and enforce equitably environmental and consumer laws. *Journal of Urban Health,* 86, no. 6: 819–824.

Oldham, J. (2011, August 22). Demand for locally grown produce spurs rise of urban farms. *Boston Globe*, p. A4.

Oliver, J. E. (2005). *The making of an American epidemic.* New York: Oxford University Press.

Oliver, J. E. (2006). *Fat politics: The real story behind America's obesity epidemic.* New York: Oxford University Press.

Olveea, N. N., Knox, B., Scherer, R., Maldonado, G., Sharma, S. V., Alastuey, L., and Bush, J. A. (2008). A healthy lifestyle program for Latino daughters and mothers: The BOUNCE overview and process evaluation. *American Journal of Health Education*, 39, no. 5: 283–295.

O'Neill, K., Williams, K. J., and Reznik, V. (2008). Engaging Latino residents to build a healthier community in Mid-City San Diego. *American Journal of Preventive Medicine*, 34, no. 3: S36–S41.

Opalinski, A. (2010). Key factors in Haitian and Hispanic children and obesity: Parent answers. *Journal for Nurse Practitioners*, 6, no. 4: 281–286.

Orbach, S. (2006). Commentary: There is a public health crisis—it's not fat on the body but fat in the mind and the fat of profits. *International Journal of Epidemiology*, 35, no. 1: 67–69.

Orsini, N. (2010). Social media: How home health care agencies can join the chorus of empowered voices. *Home Health Care Management*, 22, no. 3: 213–217.

Osel-Assibey, G., Kyrou, I., Adi, Y., Kumar, S., and Matyka, K. (2010). Dietary and lifestyle interventions for weight management in adults from minority ethnic/non-white groups: A systematic review. *Obesity Reviews*, 11, no. 1: 768–776.

Ostbye, T., Dement, J. M., and Krause, K. M. (2007). Obesity and workers' compensation: Results from the Duke Health and Safety Surveillance System. *Archives of Internal Medicine*, 167, no. 8: 766–773.

Papas, M. A., Alberg, A. J., Ewing, R., Helzlsouer, K. J., Gary, T. L., and Lassen, A. C. (2007). The built environment and obesity. *Epidemiologic Reviews*, 29, no. 1: 129–143.

Paradis, E. (2010). *Changing meaning of fat: Fat, obesity, epidemics, and America's children.* Unpublished doctoral dissertation, Stanford University, School of Education.

Parikh, N. I., Pencina, M. J., Wang, T. J., Lanier, K. J., Fox, C. S., D'Agostino, R. B., and Vasan, R. S. (2008). Increasing trends in incidence of overweight and obesity over 5 decades. *American Journal of Medicine*, 120, no. 3: 242–250.

Parker-Pope, T. (2008, March 31). Fat bias worse for women. *New York Times*, p. A23.

Parker-Pope, T. (2011a, March 31). Fat stigma is spreading around the globe. *New York Times*, pp. A1, A3.

Parker-Pope, T. (2011b, May 17). Taking measure of weight-loss plans, and the studies of them. *New York Times*, p. D5.

Passel, J., Cohn, D., and Lopez, M. (2011). *Hispanics account for more than half of nation's growth in the past decade*. Washington, DC: Pew Hispanic Center.

Pearce, J., and Day, P. (2010). Neighbourhood histories and health: Social deprivation and food retailing in Christchurch, New Zealand, 1966–2005. In A. A. Lake, T. G. Townshend, and S. Alvanides (Eds.), *Obesogenic environments: Complexities, perceptions, and objective measures* (pp. 183–198). Oxford, UK: Blackwell Publishing.

Pearsall, H., and Pierce, J. (2010). Urban sustainability and environmental justice: Evaluating the linkages in public planning/policy discourse. *Local Environment*, 15, no. 6: 569–580.

Peltz, G., Aguirre, M. T., Sanderson, M., and Fadden, M. K. (2010). The role of fat mass index in determining obesity. *American Journal of Human Biology*, 22, no. 5: 639–647.

Perdue, W. C., Stone, L. A., and Gostin, L. O. (2003). The built environment and its relationship to the public's health: The legal framework. *American Journal of Public Health*, 93, no. 9: 1390–1394.

Perez-Escamilla, R. (2011). Acculturation, nutrition, and health disparities in Latinos. *American Journal of Clinical Nutrition*, 93, no. 5: 1163S–1167S.

Perkins, F. (2009). A rights-based approach to assessing health determinates. *Global Health Promotion*, 16, no. 1: 61–64.

Peters, J., Ellis, E., Goyder, E., and Blank, L. (2005). Obesity: Tackling the problem at the community level. *Human Ecology*, Special Issue, 13, no. 1: 11–15.

Petersen, M. (2007). Economic costs of diabetes in the United States in 2007. *Diabetes Care*, 31, no. 3: 596–615.

Pezzullo, P. C., and Sandler, R. (2007). Introduction: Revisiting the environmental justice challenge to environmentalism. In R. Sandler and P. C. Pezzullo (Eds.), *Environmental justice and environmentalism: The social justice challenge to the environmental movement* (pp. 1–24). Cambridge, MA: MIT Press.

Phelan, S. (2009). Obesity in minority women: Calories, commerce, and culture. *Obstetrics and Gynecology Clinics in North America*, 36, no. 2: 379–392.

Phelan, S., Butryn, M., and Wing, R. R. (2007). Obesity prevention during adulthood. In S. Kumanyika and R. C. Brownson (Eds.), *Handbook of obesity prevention: A resource for health professionals* (pp. 489–514). New York: Springer.

Philipson, T. J., and Posner, R. A. (2008). Is the obesity epidemic a public health problem? A review of Zoltan J. Acs and Alan Lyles's *Obesity, Business, and Public Policy. Journal of Economic Literature*, 46, no. 4: 974–982.

Philpott, T. (2010, April 20). Time for the public to reinvest in food-system infrastructure. *Grist*. http://www.grist.org/article/2010–04-time-for-the-public-to-invest-in-food-system-infrastructure. Accessed 9/10/10.

Pinstrup-Andersen. P. (2009). Food security: Definition and measurement. *Food Security*, 1, no. 1: 5–7.

Pirie, G. H. (1983). On spatial justice. *Environment and Planning*, 15, no. 4: 465–473.

Pomeranz, J. L. (2008). A historical analysis of public health, the law, and stigmatized social groups: The need for both overweight and weight bias legislation. *Obesity*, 16, no. 1: S93–S103.

Pomeranz, J. L., and Brownell, K. D. (2008). Legal and public health considerations affecting the success, reach, and impact of menu-labeling laws. *American Journal of Public Health*, 98, no. 9: 1578–1583.

Popkin, B. M. (2007). Global context of obesity. In S. Kumanyika and R. C. Brownson (Eds.), *Handbook of obesity prevention: A resource for health professionals* (pp. 227–238). New York: Springer.

Pothukuchi, K. (2004). Community food assessment: A first step in planning for community food security. *Journal of Planning Education and Research*, 23, no. 4: 356–377.

Pothukuchi, K., Joseph, H., Burton, H., and Fisher, A. (2002). *What's cooking in your food system?* Venice, CA: Community Food Security Coalition.

Pouliou, T., and Elliott, S. J. (2009). Individual and socio-environmental determinates of overweight and obesity in Canada. *Health Place*, 16, no. 2: 389–398.

Powarka, L. R., Kaczyski, A. T., and Flack, A. I. (2008). Place to play: Association of park space and facilities with healthy weight status among children. *Journal of Community Health*, 33, no. 5: 344–350.

Powell, L. A., Williamson, J. B., and Branco, K. J. (1996). *The senior rights movement: Framing the policy debate in America.* New York: Twayne Publishers.

Powell, L. M., Auld, M. C., Chaloupka, F. J., O'Malley, P. M., and Johnston, L. D. (2007). Associations between access to food stores and adolescent body mass index. *American Journal of Preventive Medicine*, 33, no. 4: 301–307.

Powell, L. M., Ham, E., and Chaloupka, F. J. (2010). Economic contextual factors, food consumption, and obesity among U.S. adolescents. *Journal of Nutrition*, 140, no. 6: 1175–1180.

Powell, L. M., Slater, S., Mirtcheva, D., Bao, Y., and Chaloupka, F. J. (2007). Food store availability and neighborhood characteristics in the United States. *Preventive Medicine*, 44:189–195.

Powers, M., and Faden, R. (2006). *Social justice: The moral foundation of public health and health policy.* New York: Oxford University Press.

Prendergast, S. (2010). *Community gardens and urban agriculture: Reclaiming the market place.* Senior Project. California Polytechnic State University.

Prentice, A. M. (2006). The emerging epidemic of obesity in developing countries. *International Journal of Epidemiology*, 35, no. 1: 93–99.

Preskill, H., and Catambas, T. T. (2006). *Reframing evaluation through appreciative inquiry.* Thousand Oaks, CA: Sage Publications.

Pretty, J., Peacock, J., Sellens, M., and Griffin, M. (2005). The mental and physical health outcomes of green exercise. *International Journal of Environmental Health Research*, 15, no. 5: 319–337,

Prince, S, A Jnnsoch, I., and Tranmer, J. E. (2008). Self-measured waist circumference in older patients with heart failure: A study of validity and reliability using a Myo Tape (R). *Journal of Cardiopulmonary Rehabilitation and Prevention*, 28, no. 1: 43–47.

Project CAFÉ. (2007). *Food access in Central and South Los Angeles: Mapping injustice, agenda for action.* Los Angeles: Center for Food and Justice.

Pudup, M. B. (2008). It takes a garden: Cultivating citizen-subjects in organized garden projects. *Geoforum*, 39, no. 3: 1228–1240.

Puhl, R. M., and Heuer, C. A. (2009). The stigma of obesity: A review and update. *Obesity*, 17, no. 5: 941–964.

Puhl, R. M., and Heuer, C. A. (2010). Obesity stigma: Important considerations for public health. *American Journal of Public Health*, 100, no. 6: 1019–1028.

Rains, J. W., and Ray, D. W. (2007). Participatory action research for community health promotion, *Public Health Nursing*, 12, no. 4: 256–261.

Raloff, J. (2010, August 16). The high cost of diabetes. *ScienceNews.com*. Accessed 12/28/11.

Raphael, D. (2006). Social determinants of health: Present status, unanswered questions, and future directions. *International Journal of Health Services*, 36, no. 4: 651–677.

Records, K., Keller, C., Ainsworth, B., and Permana, P. A. (2008). Overweight and obesity in postpartum Hispanic women. *Health Care for Women International*, 29, no. 6: 649–667.

Redman, N., Baer, H. J., and Hicks, L. S. (2011). Health behaviors and racial disparity in blood pressure control in the National Health and Nutrition Examination Survey. *Hypertension*, 57, no. 4: 383–389.

Reed, D. F. (2004). *Literacy for environmental justice: Youth Envision's Good Neighbor Project in Bayview Hunters Point: A case study.* San Francisco: Youth Envision.

Reifsnider, E., Hargraves, M., Williams, K. J., Cooks, J., and Hall, V. (2010). Shaking and rattling: Developing a child obesity prevention program using a faith-based community approach. *Family and Community Health*, 33, no. 2: 144–151.

Reinehr, T., Dobe, M., Winkel, K., Schaefer, A., and Hoffman, D. (2010). Obesity in disabled children and adolescents: An overlooked group of patients. *Deutsches Arzteblatt International*, 107, no. 15: 268–275.

Reininger, B. M., Barroso, C. S., Mitchell-Bennett, L., Cantu, E., Fernandez, M. E., Gonzalez, D. A., Chavez, M., Freeberg, D., and McAlister, A. (2010). Process evaluation and participatory methods in an obesity-prevention media campaign for Mexican Americans. *Health Promotion Practice*, 11, no. 3: 347–357.

Renzaho, A. M. N., and Mellow, D. (2010). Food security measurement in cultural pluralism: Missing the point or conceptual misunderstanding? *Nutrition*, 26, no. 1: 1–9.

Reynolds, K., Gu, D., Whelton, P. K., Wu, X., Duan, X., Mo, J., and He, J. (2007). *Obesity*, 15, no. 1: 10–18.

Reynolds, L. T. (2004). The globalization of the organic agro-food networks. *World Development*, 32, no. 5: 725–743.

Reynolds, S. L., Saito, Y., and Crimmins, E. M. (2005). The impact of obesity on active life expectancy in older American men and women. *Gerontologist*, 45, no. 4: 438–444.

Rhoden, J. (2002). Growing healthy communities through urban gardening. *New Life Journal*, 3, no. 5: 1–3.

Rhodes, E. L. (2003). *Environmental justice in America: A new paradigm*. Bloomington: University of Indiana Press.

Rich, E., Monaghan, L. F., and Aphramor, L. (Eds.). (2011). *Debating obesity: Critical perspectives*. New York: Palgrave Macmillan.

Richardson, J. (2009, March 28). *The food justice movement ignored*. Change.org.

Richardson, L. D., and Norris, M. (2010). Access to health and health care: How race and ethnicity matter. *Mount Sinai Journal of Medicine*, 77, no. 2: 166–177.

Richtel, M. (2011, April 21). In online games, a path to young consumers. *New York Times*, pp. A1, A15.

Rifkin, G. (2011, May 19). Cash crops under glass and up on the roof. *New York Times*, p. B5.

Rigby, N. (2006). Commentary: Counterpoint to Campos et al. *International Journal of Epidemiology*, 35, no. 1: 79–80.

Robbins, L. (2011, April 6). If the meal is fatty and salty, a proposal would take the toys away. *New York Times*, p. A19.

Robert, S. A., and Reither, E. N. (2004). A multilevel analysis of race, community disadvantage, and body mass index among adults in the U.S. *Social Science and Medicine*, 59, no. 2: 2421–2434.

Roberts, P. (2008). *The end of food*. New York: Houghton Mifflin.

Robertson, A., Brunner, E., and Sheiham, A, (2006). Food is a political issue. In M. Marmot and R. G. Robertson (Eds.), *Social determinants of health* (pp. 172–195). New York: Oxford University Press.

Robertson, C. (2011, August 22). Preaching a healthy diet in the deep-fried delta. *New York Times*, pp. A1, A3.

Robertson-Wilson, J., and Giles-Corti. B. (2010). Walkability, neighborhood design, and obesity. In A. A. Lake, T. G. Townshend, and S. Alvanides (Eds.), *Obesogenic environments: Complexities, perceptions, and objective measures* (pp. 21–39). Oxford, UK: Blackwell Publishing.

Robert Wood Johnson Foundation. (2010). *School policies and practices to improve health and prevent obesity: National Elementary School Survey Results, "Bridging the Gap."* Princeton, N.J.: Author.

Rootes, C., and Saunders, C. (2008). *The development of the global justice movement in Britain*. Canterbury, England: University of Kent at Canterbury.

Rosai, M. C., Borg, A., Bodenios, J. S., Tellez, T., and Ockene, I. S. (2011). Awareness of diabetes risk factors and prevention strategies among a sample of low-income Latinos with no known diagnosis of diabetes. *Diabetes Education*, 37, no. 1: 47–55.

Rose, D., Bodor, N., Hutchinson, P. L., and Swalm, C. M. (2010). The importance of a multi-dimensional approach for studying the links between food access and consumption. *Journal of Nutrition*, 140, no. 5: 1170–1174.

Ross, R., Berentzer, T., Bradshaw, A. J., Janssen, I., Kahn, H. S., Katzmarzyk, P. T., Kuk, J. L., Seidell, J. C., Snyder, M. B., Sarensen, I. A., and Despres, J. P. (2008). Does the relationship between waist circumference and mortality depend on measurement protocol for waist circumference? *Obesity Reviews*, 9, no. 4: 312–325.

Rotegard, A. K., Moore, S. M., Fagermoen, M. S., and Rutland, C. M. (2010). Health assets: A concept analysis. *Nursing Studies*, 47, no. 4: 513–525.

Rothman, K. J. (2008). BMI-related errors in the measurement of obesity. *International Journal of Obesity*, 32, suppl. 3: S56–S59.

Rowlands, I., Graves, N., de Jersey, S., McIntyre, H. D., and Callaway, L. (2010). Obesity in pregnancy: Outcomes and economics. *Seminars in Fetal and Neonatal Medicine*, 15, no. 2: 94–99.

Royle, T. (2010). "Low-road Americanization" and the global "McJob": A longitudinal analysis of work, pay, and unionization in the international fast-food industry. *Labor History*, 51, no. 2: 249–270.

Rueda-Clausen, C. F., Silva, F. A., and Lopez-Jaramillo, P. (2008). Epidemic of overweight and obesity in Latin America and the Caribbean. *International Journal of Cardiology*, 125, no. 1: 111–112.

Ruge, J. P. (2010). *Health and social justice*. New York: Oxford University Press.

Rundle, A., Roux, A. V. D., Freeman, L. M., Miller, D., Neckerman, K. M., and Weiss, C. C. (2007). The urban built environment and obesity in New York City: A multilevel analysis. *Health Promotion*, 21, no. 4, suppl.: 326–334.

Rush, C. E., Freitas, I., and Plank, L. D. (2009). Body size, body composition, and fat distribution: Comparative analysis of European, Maori, Pacific Island, and Asian Indian adults. *British Journal of Nutrition*, 102:632–641.

Russell-Mayhew, S. (2006). Eating disorders and obesity as social justice issues: Implications for research and practice. *Journal of Social Action in Counseling and Psychology*, 1, no. 1: 1–13.

Ryan, W. (1971). *Blaming the victim*. New York: Random House.

Sacks, G., Swinburn, B., and Lawrence, M. (2009). Obesity policy action framework and analysis grids for a comprehensive policy approach to reducing obesity. *Obesity Reviews*, 10, no. 1: 76–86.

Saguy, A. C. (2005). "Obesity epidemic" overblown, conclude UCLA sociologists. *UCLA College of Letters and Science: News about the College*. http://www.college.ucla.edu/news/05/obesitystudy.html. Accessed 9/1/10.

Saguy, A. C., and Almeling, R. (2008). Fat in the fire? Science, the news media, and the "Obesity Epidemic." *Sociological Forum*, 23, no. 1: 53–83.

Saldivar-Tanaka, L., and Krasny, M. E. (2004). Culturing community development, neighborhood open space, and civic agriculture: The case of Latino community gardens in New York City. *Agriculture and Human Values*, 21, no. 4: 399–412.

Sallis, J. F., and Glanz, K. (2009). Physical activity and food environments: Solutions to the obesity epidemic. *Milbank Quarterly*, 87, no. 1: 123–154.

Samuels, S. E., Craypo, L., Lawrence, S., Lingas, E. O., and Dorfman, L. (2007). Media, marketing and advertising and obesity. In S. Kumanyika and R. C. Brownson (Eds.), *Handbook of obesity prevention: A resource for health professionals* (pp. 209–226). New York: Springer.

Sanjek, R. (2009). *Gray Panthers*. Philadelphia: University of Pennsylvania Press.

Satia-Abouta, J. (2003). Dietary acculturation: Definition, process, assessment, and implications. *International Journal of Human Ecology*, 4, no. 1: 71–86.

Scharoun-Lee, M., Kaufman, J. S., Popkin, B. M., and Gordon-Larsen, P. (2009). Obesity, race/ethnicity, and life course socioeconomic status across the transition from adolescence to adulthood. *Journal of Epidemiology Community Health*, 63, no. 2: 133–139.

Schild, D. R., and Sable, M. R. (2006). Public health and social work. In S. Gehlert and T. A. Browne (Eds.), *Handbook of health social work* (pp. 70–122). New York: John Wiley and Sons.

Schlosberg, D. (2007). *Defining environmental justice: Theories, movements, and nature*. New York: Oxford University Press.

Schlosser, E. (1998a, September 3). Fast-food nation: Meat and potatoes. Part One. *Rolling Stone Magazine*. http://www.mespotlight.org/media/press/rollingston2 .html. Accessed 4/7/11.

Schlosser, E. (1998b, September 3). Fast-food nation: The true cost of America's diet. Part Two. *Rolling Stone Magazine*. http://www.mespotlight.org/media/press/ rollingston2.html. Accessed 4/7/11.

Schlosser, E. (2005). *Fast food nation: The dark side of the all-American meal*. New York: Harper Perennial.

Schmitt, N. M., Wagner, N., and Kirch, W. (2007). Consumers' freedom of choice: Advertising aimed at children, product placement, and food labeling. *Journal of Public Health*, 15, no. 1: 57–62.

Schwartz, M. B., and Brownell, K. D. (2007). Actions necessary to prevent childhood obesity: Creating the climate for change. *Journal of Law, Medicine, and Ethics*, 35, no. 1: 78–89.

Schwartz, M. B., Chambliss, H. O., Brownell, K. D., Blair, S. N., and Billington, C. (2003). Weight bias among health professionals specializing in obesity. *Obesity Research*, 11, no. 10: 1033–1039.

Schwimmer, J. B. (2005). Review: Preventing childhood obesity. *Environmental Health Perspective*, 113, p. A706.

ScienceDaily. (2007, August 30). Zip Codes and property values predict obesity rates. Author. http://www.sciencedaily.com/releases/2007/081070829090143 .htm. Accessed 8/31/10.

ScienceDaily. (2009, August 12). Food stamp use linked to weight gain, study finds, pp. 1–3.

Seghers, J., and Claessens, A. L. (2010). Bias in self-reported height and weight in preadolescence. *Journal of Pediatrics*, 157, no. 6: 911–916.

Seidell, J. C. (2000). Obesity, insulin resistance, and diabetes—a worldwide epidemic. *British Journal of Nutrition*, 83, suppl. 1: 55–58.

Seifer, S. D. (2006). Building and sustaining community-institutional partnerships for prevention research: Findings from a national collaborative. *Journal of Urban Health*, 83, no. 6: 989–1003.

Seo, D.-C., and Sa, J. (2007). A meta-analysis of psycho-behavioral obesity interventions among U.S. multiethnic and minority adults. *Preventive Medicine*, 47, no. 6: 573–582.

Severance, J. H., and Zinnah, S. L. (2011). Community-based perceptions of neighborhood health in urban neighborhoods. *Journal of Community Health Nursing*, 26, no. 1: 14–23.

Severson, K. (2008, August 12). Los Angeles stages a fast food intervention. *New York Times*, p. A18.

Shama, M. (2008). Physical activity interventions in Hispanic American girls and women. *Obesity Reviews*, 9, no. 6: 560–571.

Sherman, R. F. (2004). The promise of youth is in the present. *National Civic Review*, 93, no. 1: 50–55.

Sherry, B., Jefferds, M. E., and Grummer-Strawn, M. L. (2007). Accuracy of adolescent self-report of height and weight in assessing overweight status: A literature review. *Archives of Pediatrics and Adolescent Medicine*, 161, no. 12: 1154–1161.

Shields, M., Gorber, S. C., and Tremblay, M. S. (2008). *Estimates of obesity based on self-report versus direct measures*. Health Reports, Ottawa: Statistics Canada.

Shimakawa, T., Sarlie, P., Carpenter, M., Dennis, B., Tell, G., Watson, R., and Williams, O. (1994). Dietary intake patterns and socioeconomic factors in the Atherosclerosis Risk in Communities Study. *Preventive Medicine*, 23, no. 4: 257–263.

Siegel, M. (2002). Antismoking advertising: Figuring out what works. *Journal of Health Communication*, 7, no. 2: 157–162.

Simen-Kapeu, A., and Veugelers, P. J. (2010). Should public health interventions aimed at reducing childhood overweight and obesity be gender-focused? *BMHC Public Health*, 10, 1–7.

Simon, M. (2006a). *Appetite for profit: How the food industry undermines our health and how to fight back*. New York: Nation Books.

Simon, M. (2006b). Can food companies be trusted to self-regulate? An analysis of corporate lobbying and deception to undermine children's health. *Loyola L.A.L. Review*, 169–236.

Sims, R., Gordon, S., Garcia, W., Clark, E., Monye, D., Callender, C., and Campbell, A. (2008). Perceived stress and eating behaviors in a community-based sample of African Americans. *Eating Behaviors*, 9, no. 2: 137–142.

Singer, N. (2011, May 15). Foods with benefits, or so they say. Sunday Business, *New York Times*, pp. 1, 6.

Singh, G. K., Kogan, M. D., Van Dyck, P. C., and Siashpush, M. (2008). Racial/ethnic, socioeconomic, and behavioral determinants of childhood and adolescent obesity in the United States: Analyzing independent and joint associations. *Annals of Epidemiology*, 18, no. 9: 682–695.

Skelton, J. A., Cook, S. R., Auinger, P., Klein, J. D., and Barlow, S. E. (2009). Prevalence and trends of severe obesity among U.S. children and adults. *Academic Pediatrics*, 9, no. 5: 322–329.

Slusser, W. M., Cumberland, W. G., Browdy, B. L., Winham, D. M., and Neumann, C. G. (2005). Overweight in urban, low-income, African American and Hispanic children attending Los Angeles elementary schools: Research stimulating action. *Public Health Nutrition*, 8, no. 2: 141–148.

Smit, J., Ratta, A., and Nasr, J. (1996). *Urban agriculture, food, jobs, and sustainable cities*. New York: United Nations Development Programme.

Smith, A. F. (2009). *Eating history: 30 turning points in the making of American cuisine*. New York: Columbia University Press.

Smith, J. C. (1999). *Understanding childhood obesity*. Jackson: University of Mississippi Press.

Smith, L. H. (2010). Piloting the use of teen mentors to promote a healthy diet and physical activity among children in Australia. *Journal of Specialists in Pediatric Nursing*, 16, no. 1: 16–28.

Smith, M. C. (2009). Obesity as a social problem in the United States: Application of the public arenas model. *Policy Politics and Nursing Practice*, 10, no. 2: 134–142.

Smith, S. (2008). From the farm to the city: Using agricultural supplies to irrigate urban landscapes. *Journal AWWA*, 100, no. 5: 96–100.

Soja, E. W. (2010). *Seeking spatial justice*. Minneapolis: University of Minnesota Press.

Solovay, S. (2000). *Tipping the scales of justice: Fighting weight-based discrimination*. Amherst, NY: Prometheus Books.

Sommers, A. R. (2009). *Obesity among older Americans*. Washington, DC: Congressional Research Office.

Song, H.-J., Gittelsohn, J., Kim, M., Suratkar, S., Sharma, S., and Anliker, J. (2010). Korean American storeowners' perceived barriers and motivators for implementing a corner store-based program. *Health Promotion Practice*, 12, no. 3: 472–482.

Sothern, M. S., Myers, V. H., and Martin, P. D. (2004). *Effectiveness of interventions for overweight and obesity in children and adults*. Baton Rouge, LA: Pennington Biomedical Research Center.

Spear, B., Barlow, S. E., Ervin, C., Ludwig, D. S., Saelens, B., Schetzina, K. E., and Taveras, E. M. (2007). Recommendations for treatment of child and adolescent overweight and obesity. *Pediatrics*, 120, suppl.: S254–S288.

Spruijt-Metz, D. (2011). Etiology, treatment, and prevention of obesity in childhood and adolescence: A decade in review. *Journal of Research on Adolescence*, 21, no. 1: 129–152.

Srinivasan, S., Liam, R., O'Fallon, L. R., and Dearry, A. (2003). Creating healthy communities, healthy homes, healthy people: Initiating a research agenda on the built environment and public health. *American Journal of Public Health*, 93, no. 9: 1446–1450.

Stanley, A. (2009). Just space or spatial justice? Difference, discourse, and environmental justice. *Local Environment*, 14, no. 10: 999–1014.

Steele, C. (2008). *Hungry city.* London: Chatto and Windos.

Stettler, N. (2007). Obesity risk factors and prevention in early life: Pre-gestation through infancy. In S. Kumanyika and R. C. Brownson (Eds.), *Handbook of obesity prevention: A resource for health professionals* (pp. 404–428). New York: Springer.

Stewart, R. S., and Korol, S. A. (2010). Designing fat: Re-constructing the global obesity epidemic. *International Journal of Applied Philosophy*, 23, no. 2: 285–304.

Stodolska, M., and Shinew, K. J. (2010). Environmental constraints on leisure time physical activity among Latino urban residents. *Qualitative Research in Sport, Exercise, and Health*, 2, no. 3: 313–335.

Stokols, B. A., Green, L. W., Leischow, S., Holmes, B., and Buchholz, K. (2003). An integrative framework for community partnering to translate theory into effective health promotion strategy. *American Journal of Health Promotion*, 18, no. 2: 168–176.

Stolberg, S. G., and Neuman, W. (2011, February 7). Restaurant nutrition draws focus of first lady: Expanding the push for healthier eating. *New York Times*, pp. A11, A13.

Stommel, M., and Schoenborn, C. A. (2010). Variations in BMI and prevalence of health risks in diverse racial and ethnic populations. *Obesity.* doi:10.1038/oby .2009.472.

Story, M., Kaphingst, K. M., Robinson-O'Brien, R., and Glanz, K. (2008). Creating healthy food and eating environments: Policy and environmental approaches. *Annual Review of Public Health*, 29:253–271.

Striffler, S. (2005). *Chicken: The dangerous transformation of America's favorite food.* New Haven, CT: Yale University Press.

Strine, T. W., Makdad, A. H., Dube, S. R., Balluz, L., Gonzalez, O., Berry, J. T., Manderscheid, R., and Kroen, K. (2008). The association of depression and anxiety with obesity and unhealthy behaviors. *General Hospital Psychiatry*, 30, no. 2: 127–137.

Strum, R. (2007). Increases in morbid obesity in the USA: 2000–2005. *Public Health*, 121, no. 7: 492–496.

Strum, R., and Cohen, D. A. (2009). Zoning for health? The year-old ban on new fast-food restaurants in South LA. *Health Affairs*, 28, no. 6: 1088–1097.

Studenski, S., Perera, S., Hile, E., Keller, V., Spadola-Bogard, J., and Garcia, J. (2010). Interactive video dance games for healthy older adults. *Journal of Nutrition, Health, and Aging*, 14, no. 10: 850–852.

Suarez-Balcazar, Y., and Harper, G. (Eds.). (2004). *Empowerment and participatory evaluation in community intervention: Multiple benefits.* New York: Haworth Press.

Suarez-Balcazar, Y., Hellwig, M., Kouba, J., Redmond, L., Martinez, L., Block, D., Kohrman, C., and Peterman, W. (2006). The making of an interdisciplinary partnership: The case of the Chicago Food System Collaborative. *American Journal of Community Psychology*, 38, nos. 1–2: 113–123.

Suarez-Balcazar, Y., Redmond, L., Kouba, J., Hellwig, M., Davis, R., Martinez, L. I., and Jones, L. (2007). Introducing systems of change in the schools: The case of school luncheons and vending machines. *American Journal of Community Psychology*, 39, nos. 3–4: 335–345.

Sui, D. Z. (2003). Musings on the fat city: Are obesity and urban forms linked? *Urban Geography*, 24, no. 1: 75–84.

Surgeon General. (2001). *A Surgeon General's Call to Action to Prevent and Reduce Overweight and Obesity*. Washington, DC: Department of Health and Human Services.

Surgeon General. (2007). *A Surgeon General's Call to Action to Prevent and Reduce Overweight and Obesity*. Washington, DC: Department of Health and Human Services.

Sutton, E. (2005). *Obesity, poverty, and the case for community supported agriculture in New York State*. New York: Hunger Action Network of New York State.

Sutton, S. E. (2007). A social justice perspective on youth and community development: Theorizing the process and outcomes of partner. *Children, Youth, and Environment*, 17, no. 2: 1–30.

Sweeting, H. (2011). "No admittance to obese persons." *Journal of Epidemiology and Community Health*, 65, no. 4: 386.

Swinburn, B., Gill, T., and Kumanyika, S. (2005). Obesity prevention: A proposed framework for translating evidence into action. *Obesity Review*, 6, no. 1: 23–33.

Swinburn, B. A., Caterson, I., Seidell, J. C., and James, W. P. T. (2004). Diet, nutrition, and the prevention of excess weight and obesity. *Public Health Nutrition*, 7, no. 2: 123–146.

Swinburn, B. A., Egger, G., and Raza, F. (1999). Dissecting obesogenic environments: The development and application of a framework for identifying and prioritizing environmental interventions for obesity. *Preventive Medicine*, 29, no. 6: 563–570.

Syme, S. L. (2008). Reducing racial and social-class inequalities in health: The need for a new approach. *Health Affairs*, 27, no. 2: 456–459.

Sze, J. (2004). Asian American activism for environmental justice. *Peace Review*, 16, no. 2: 149–156.

Sze, J. (2007). *Noxious New York: The racial politics of urban health and environmental justice*. Cambridge, MA: MIT Press.

Sze, J., and London, J. K. (2008). Environmental justice at the crossroads. *Sociological Compass*, 2, no. 4: 1331–1354.

Talwar, J. P. (2002). *Fast food, fast track: Immigrants, big business, and the American dream*. Boulder, CO: Westview Press.

Tavernise, S. (2011a, February 5). In census, minorities show gains in youth. *New York Times*, p. A10.

Tavernise, S. (2011b, April 6). Numbers of children of whites falling fast. *New York Times*, p. A14.

Tavernise, S. (2011c, September 9). Vegetable gardens are booming in a fallow economy. *New York Times*, pp. A13–A14.

Taylor, D. E. (2000). The rise of the environmental justice paradigm: Injustice framing and the social construction of environmental discourses. *American Behavioral Scientist*, 43, no. 4: 508–580.

Taylor, G. (2002). *Building the case for the prevention of chronic disease*. Winnipeg, Manitoba, Canada: University of Manitoba.

Taylor, J. (2009). Fear of failure: A childhood epidemic. Keep Kids Healthy.com.

Taylor, W. C., Carlos Poston, W. S., Jones, L., and Kraft, M. K. (2006). Environmental justice: Obesity, physical activity, and healthy eating. *Journal of Physical Activity and Health*, 3, no. 1: S30–S54.

Taylor, W. C., Floyd, M. F., Whitt-Glover, M. C., and Brooks, J. (2007). A framework for collaboration between the public health and parks and recreation fields to study disparities in physical activity. *Journal of Physical Activity and Health*, 4, suppl.: S50–S63.

Taylor, W. C., Hepworth, J. T., Lees, E., Feliz, K., Ahsan, S., Cassells, A., Volding, D. C., and Tobin, J. N. (2008). Obesity, physical activity, and the environment: Is there a legal basis for environmental justice? *Environmental Justice*, 1, no. 1: 45–48.

Ten Eyck, T. A. (2007). Public opinion and obesity: A different look at a modern-day epidemic. In H. D. Davies and H. E. Fitzgerald (Eds.), *Obesity in childhood and adolescence* (pp. 183–198). Westport, CT: Praeger.

Teran, L. M., Belkin, K. L., and Johnson, C. A. (2002). An exploration of psychosocial determinants of obesity among Hispanic women. *Hispanic Journal of Behavioral Sciences*, 24, no. 1: 92–103.

Teufel-Shone, N. I. (2006). Promising strategies for obesity prevention and treatment within American Indiana communities. *Journal of Transcultural Nursing*, 17, no. 3: 224–229.

Thompson, J. L. (2008). Obesity and consequent health risks: Is prevention realistic and achievable? *Archives of Disease in Childhood*, 93, no. 9: 722–724.

Tolbert, R., Brooks-Gunn, J., and McLanahan, S. (2007). Racial and ethnic differentials in overweight and obesity among 3-year-old children. *American Journal of Public Health*, 97, no. 2: 298–305.

Torre, M., and Fine, M. (2005). Researching and resisting: Democratic policy research by and for youth. In S. Ginwright, P. Noguera, and J. Cammarota (Eds.), *Beyond resistance: Youth activism and community change* (pp. 269–285). New York: Routledge.

Townsend, M. S. (2006). Obesity in low-income communities: Prevalence, effects, a place to begin. *Journal of the American Dietetic Association*, 106, no. 1: 34–37.

Townshend, T. G., Ells, L., Alvanides, S., and Lake, A. A. (2010). Towards transdisciplinary approaches to tackle obesity. In A. A. Lake, T. G. Townshend, and

S. Alvanides (Eds.), *Obesogenic environments: Complexities, perceptions, and objective measures* (pp. 11–20). Oxford, UK: Blackwell Publishing.

Travaline, K. A. (2008). *Urban agriculture: Enhancing food democracy in Philadelphia*. Philadelphia: Drexel University.

Trent, M., Jennings, J. M., Waterfield, G., Lyman, L. M., and Thomas, H. (2009). Finding targets for obesity intervention in urban communities: School-based health centers and the interface with affected youth. *Journal of Urban Health*, 86, no. 4: 571–583.

Treuhaft, S., and Karpyn, A. (2011). *The grocery gap: Who has access to healthy food and why it matters*. Philadelphia: The Food Trust.

Trimbal, B., and Morgenstern, L. B. (2008). Stroke in minorities. *Neurologic Clinics*, 26, no. 4: 1177–1190.

Trogdon, J. G., Finkelstein, E. A., Hylands, T., Dellea, S. J., and Kamal-Bahl, S. J. (2008). Indirect costs of obesity: A review of the literature. *Obesity Reviews*, 9, no. 5: 489–500.

Tschamier, J. M., Conn, K. M., Cook, S. R., and Halterman, J. S. (2009). Underestimation of children's weight status: Views of parents in an urban community. *Clinical Pediatrics*, 49, no. 5: 470–476.

Twiss, J., Dickinson, J., Duma, S., Kleinman, T., Paulsen, H., and Rilveria, L. (2003). Community gardens: Lessons learned from California healthy cities and communities. *American Journal of Public Health*, 93, no. 9: 1435–1438.

Ulijaszek, S. J. (2008). Seven models of population obesity. *Angiology*, 59, suppl. 2: 34S–38S.

United Food and Commercial Workers Union. (2010a, August 31). Ending Walmart's rural stranglehold. http://www.foodfirst.org/en/node/3076. Accessed 9/10/10.

United Food and Commercial Workers Union. (2010b, August 31). Food first. http://www.foodfirst.org/en/node/3076. Accessed 9/10/10.

United States Department of Agriculture. (2009). *Food security in the United States: Key statistics and graphs*. Washington, DC: Author.

United States Department of Agriculture. (2010). *Report of the Dietary Guidelines Advisory Committee on the Dietary Guidelines for America*. Washington, DC: Author.

University of Michigan. (2007). *An exploration of community coalitions as a means to address overweight and obesity*. Ann Arbor: Center for Managing Chronic Disease.

Uprising. (2008, August 20). Teens boycott fast food in their communities. www.uprising.org. Accessed 7/25/10.

Vallianatos, M. (2009). Food justice and food retail in Los Angeles. *Ecology Law Currents*, 36:186–194.

Van Baal, P. H. M., Polder, J. J., de Wit, A., Hoogenveen, R. T., Feenstra, T. L., Boshuizen, H. C., Engelfriet, P. M., and Brouwer, W. B. F. (2008). Lifetime medical costs of obesity: Prevention no cure for increasing health expenditure. *PloS Medicine*, 5, no. 2: e29–e44.

Van den Berg, A. E., and Custers, M. H. G. (2010). Gardening promotes neuroendocrine and affective restoration from stress. *Journal of Health Psychology*, 15, no. 5. doi: 10.1177/1359105310365577.

Vanderkam, L. (2010, April 19). Do food stamps feed obesity? *USA Today*, p. 2.

Van Lenthe, F. J., and Brug, J. (2010). Environmental correlates of nutrition and physical activity: Moving beyond the promise. In A. A. Lake, T. G. Townshend, and S. Alvanides (Eds.), *Obesogenic environments: Complexities, perceptions, and objective measures* (pp. 199–214). Oxford, UK: Blackwell Publishing.

Vasquez, V. B., Lanza, D., Hennessey-Lavery, S., Halpin, H. A., and Minkler, M. (2007). Addressing food security through public policy action in a community-based participatory research partnership. *Health Promotion*, 8, no. 4: 342–349.

Veenhuizen, R. V. (Ed.). (2006). *Cities farming for the future: Urban agriculture for green and productive cities*. Ottawa, Canada: International Development Research Centre.

Ver Ploeg, M., Mancino, L., and Lin, B.-H. (2006, February). Food stamps and obesity: Ironic twist or complex puzzle. *Amber News*, 1–7.

Viljoen, A. (2005). CPULs: *Continuous productive urban landscapes: Designing urban agriculture for sustainable cities*. London: Architectural Press.

Viljoen, A., and Bohn, K. (2005). Continuous productive urban landscapes: Urban agriculture as an essential infrastructure. *Urban Agriculture Magazine*, 15, no. 1: 34–36.

Viner, R., and Macfarlane, A. (2005). ABC of adolescence: Health promotion. *British Journal of Medicine*, 130:527–529.

Voicu, L., and Been, V. (2008). The effect of community gardens on neighboring property values. *Real Estate Economics*, 36, no. 2: 241–283.

Wakefield, S., Yeudall, F., Taron, C., Reynolds, J., and Skinner, A. (2007). Growing urban health: Community gardening in South-East Toronto. *Health Promotion International*, 22, no. 2: 92–101.

Walker, G. (2009). Beyond distribution and proximity: Exploring the multiple spatialities of environmental justice. *Antipode*, 41, no. 4: 614–636.

Walker, G., and Bulkeley, H. (2006). Editorial. Geographies of environmental justice. *Geoforum*, 37, no. 6: 655–659.

Walks, R. A. (2009). The urban in fragile, uncertain, neoliberal times: Towards new geographies of social justice. *Canadian Geographer / Le Géographe canadien*, 53, no. 3: 345–356.

Wallace, M. I. (2008). The spirit of environmental justice: Resurrection Hope in urban America. *Worldviews: Global Religions, Culture, and Ecology*, 12, nos. 2–3: 255–269.

Wallerstein, N., and Freudenberg, N. (1998). Linking health promotion and social justice: A rationale and two care stories. *Health Education Research*, 13, no. 3: 451–459.

Walls, H. L., Peeters, A., Proietto, J., and McNeil, J. J. (2011). Public health campaigns and obesity—a critique. *BMC Public Health*, 11:136.

Wang, Y. C., and Beydoun, M. A. (2007). The obesity epidemic in the United States— Gender, age, socioeconomic, racial/ethnic, and geographic characteristics: A systematic review and meta-regression analysis. *Epidemiologic Reviews*, 29, no. 1: 6–28.

Wang, Y. C., Beydoun, M. A., Liang, L., Caballero, B., and Kumanyika, S. K. (2008). Will all Americans become overweight or obese? Estimating the progression and cost of the U.S. obesity epidemic. *Obesity*, 16, no. 10: 2323–2330.

Wang, Y. C., Bleich, S. N., and Gortmaker, S. L. (2008). Increasing caloric contribution from sugar-sweetened beverages and 100% fruit juices among US children and adolescents, 1988–2004. *Pediatrics*, 121, no. 4: E1604–E1614.

Wang, Y. C., Gortmaker, S. L., and Traveras, E. M. (2010). Trends and racial/ethnic disparities in severe obesity among U.S. children and adolescents, 1976–2000. *International Journal of Pediatric Obesity*, 6, no. 1: 12–20.

Wang, Y. C., and Kumanyika, S. (2007). Descriptive epidemiology of obesity in the United States. In S. Kumanyika and R. C. Brownson (Eds.), *Handbook of obesity prevention: A resource for health professionals* (pp. 45–83). New York: Springer.

Wang, Y. C., and Lobstein, T. (2006). Worldwide trends in childhood overweight and obesity. *International Journal of Pediatric Obesity*, 1, no. 1: 11–25.

Wang, Z., Patterson, C. M., and Hills, A. P. (2002). A comparison of self-reported and measured height, weight, and BMI in Australian adolescents. *Australia and New Zealand Journal of Public Health*, 2, no. 5: 473–478.

Wansink, B., and Peters, J. C. (2007). The food industry role in obesity prevention. In S. Kumanyika and R. C. Brownson (Eds.), *Handbook of obesity prevention: A resource for health professionals* (pp. 193–208). New York: Springer.

Wardle, J., and Cooke, L. (2005). The impact of obesity on psychological well-being. *Clinical Endocrinology and Metabolism*, 19, no. 3: 421–440.

Warren, H. (2010). *An integrated approach to prevention of obesity in high risk families*. Lincoln: University of Nebraska.

Warren, N., Moorman, P., Dunn, M. J., Mitchell, C. S., Fisher, A., and Floyd, M. F. (2009). Southeast Raleigh minority faith-based health promotion project. *Californian Journal of Health Promotion*, 7, special issue: 87–98.

Waters, E. (2009). Building an evidence base to meet the needs of those tackling obesity prevention. *Journal of Public Health*, 31, no. 2: 300–302.

Waters, E., Ashbolt, R., Gibbs, L., Booth, M., Magarey, A., Gold, L., Lo, S. K., Gibbons, K., Green, J., O'Connor, T., Garrard, J., and Swinburn, B. (2008). Double disadvantage: The influence of ethnicity over socioeconomic position on childhood overweight and obesity: Findings from an inner urban population of primary school children. *International Journal of Pediatric Obesity*, 3, no. 4: 196–204.

Watts , R. J., and Guessous, O. (2006). Sociopolitical development: The missing link in research and policy on adolescents. In S. Ginwright, P. Noguera, and J. Cammarota (Eds.), *Beyond resistance: Youth activism and community change* (pp. 59–80). New York: Routledge.

Weeks, J. (2007). Factory farms: Are they the best way to feed the nation? *Congressional Quarterly Researcher*, 17, no. 2: 1–35.

Wekerle, G. R. (2004). Food justice movements: Policy, planning, and networks. *Journal of Planning Education and Research*, 23, no. 4: 378–386.

Wen, L. M., Orr, N., Millett, C., and Rissel, C. (2006). Driving to work and overweight and obesity: Findings from the 2003 New South Wales Health Survey, Australia. *International Journal of Obesity*, 30, no. 5: 782–786.

Whelan, E.-M., Russell, L., and Sekhar, S. (2010). *Confronting America's childhood obesity epidemic: How the health care reform law will help prevent and reduce obesity*. Washington, DC: Center for American Progress.

Whitacre, P. T., Burns, A. C., Liverman, C., and Parker, L. (2009). *Community perspectives on obesity prevention in children: Workshop summaries*. Washington, DC: National Academies Press.

Whitaker, R. C. (2006). Obesity among US urban preschool children: Relationships to race, ethnicity, and socioeconomic status. *Archives of Pediatrics and Adolescent Medicine*, 160, no. 6: 578–584.

White, M. (2007). Food access and obesity. *Obesity Reviews*, 8, suppl.1: 99–107.

White-Cooper, S., Dawkins, S. L., and Anderson, L. A. (2009). Community-institutional partnerships: Understanding trust among partners. *Health Education Behavior*, 36, no. 2: 334–347.

Whitehead, M. (2007). A typology of actions to tackle social inequalities in health. *Journal of Epidemiology of Community Health*, 61, no. 1: 473–478.

Wieringa, N. F., van der Windt, H. J., Zuiker, R. R. M., Dijkhuizen, L., Verkerk, M. A., Vonk, R. J., and Swart, J. A. A. (2008). Positioning functional foods in an ecological approach to the prevention of overweight and obesity. *Obesity Reviews*, 9, no. 4: 464–473.

Wilkins, J. L. (2007). Eating right here: Moving from concerns to food citizen. *Agriculture and Human Values*, 22, no. 3: 269–273.

Wilks, J. (2010). Child-friendly cities: A place for active citizenship in geographical and environmental education. *International Research in Geographical and Environmental Education*, 19, no. 1: 25–38.

Williams-Brown, S., Satcher, D., Alexander, W., Levine, R. S., and Gailer, M. (2007). The 100 Black Men Health Challenge: A healthy lifestyle and role model program for educated, upper-middle class, affluent African American men and their young mentees. *American Journal of Health Education*, 38, no. 1: 55–59.

Wills, J., Chinemana, F., and Rudolph, M. (2010). Growing or connecting? An urban food garden in Johannesburg. *Health Promotion International*, 25, no. 1: 33–41.

Wilson, D. (2010, July 28). A shift toward fighting fat: Antismoking efforts losing funding to a new threat. *New York Times*, pp. B1, B7.

Wilson, D. K. (2009). New perspectives on health disparities and obesity interventions in youth. *Pediatric Psychology*, 34, no. 3: 231–244.

Wilson, S., Hutson, M., and Mujahid, M. (2008). How planning and zoning contribute to inequitable development, neighborhood health, and environmental injustice. *Environmental Justice*, 1, no. 4: 211–216.

Winne, M. (2005). Education for change. *Journal of Agricultural and Environmental Ethics*, 18, no. 3: 305–310.

Winne, M. (2009). *Closing the food gap: Resetting the table in the land of plenty.* Boston: Beacon Press.

Wiseman, C. V., Gray, J. J., Mosimann, J. E., and Aherns, A. H. (1992). Cultural expectations of thinness in women: An update. *International Journal of Eating Disorders*, 11, no. 1: 85–89.

Wolch, J., Jerrett, M., Reynolds, K., McConnell, R., Chang, R., Dahmann, N., Brady, K., Gilliland, F., Su, J. G., and Berhane, K. (2011). Childhood obesity and proximity to urban parks and recreational resources: A longitudinal cohort study. *Health and Place*, 17, no. 1: 207–214.

Wolin, K. Y., and Petrelli, J. M. (2009). *Biographies of disease: Obesity.* Westport, CT: Greenwood Press.

Wong, N. T., Zimmerman, M. A., and Parker, E. A. (2010). A typology of youth participation and empowerment for children and adolescent health promotion. *American Journal of Community Psychology*, 46, nos. 1–2: 100–114.

Woodward-Lopez, G., and Flores, G. R. (2006). *Obesity in Latino communities: Prevention, principles, and action.* Sacramento: Latino Coalition for a Healthy California.

World Health Organization. (2000). *Obesity: Preventing and managing the global epidemic.* Report of a WHO consultation. WHO Technical Report Series 894. Geneva: Author.

World Health Organization. (2011). *Obesity and overweight.* Geneva: Author. http://www.who.int/mediacentre/factsheets/fs311/en/index.html. Accessed 10/25/11.

World Health Organization Expert Consultation. (2004). Appropriate body-mass index for Asian populations and its implications for policy and intervention strategies. *Lancet*, 363:157–163.

Wu, Y. (2006). Editorial. Overweight and obesity in China. *British Medical Journal*, 333:362–363.

Wyatt, S. B., Winters, K. P., and Dubbert, P. (2006). Overweight and obesity: Prevalence, consequences, and causes of a growing public health problem. *American Journal of the Medical Sciences*, 331, no. 4: 166–174.

Xie, B., Gilliland, F., Li, Y., and Rockett, H. (2003). Effects of ethnicity, family income, and education on dietary intake among adolescents. *Preventive Medicine*, 36, no. 1: 30–40.

Yach, D., Stuckler, D., and Brownell, K. D. (2006). Epidemiologic and economic consequences of the global epidemics of obesity and diabetes. *Nature Medicine*, 12, no. 1: 62–66.

Yancey, A. K., Cole, D. L., Brown, R., Williams, J. D., Hillier, A., Kline, B. S., Ashe, M., Grier, S. A., Backman, D., and McCarthy, W. J. (2009). A cross-sectional prevalence study of ethnically targeted and general audience outdoor obesity-related advertising. *Milbank Quarterly*, 87, no. 1: 155–184.

Yancey, A. K., Ory, M. G., and Davis, S. M. (2006). Dissemination of physical activity promotion interventions in underserved populations. *American Journal of Preventive Medicine*, 31, no. 4: 82–91.

Yang, Z., and Hall, A. G. (2007). The financial burden of overweight and obesity among elderly Americans: The dynamics of weight, longevity, and health care cost. *Health Services Research*, 43, no. 3: 849–868.

Yanovski, S. Z., and Yanovski, J. A. (2011, March 17). Obesity prevalence in the United States: Up, down, or sideways. *New England Journal of Medicine*, 364: 987–989.

Yeh, M.-C., Viladrich, A., Bruning, N., and Roye, C. (2008). Determinants of Latina obesity in the United States: The role of selective acculturation. *Journal of Transcultural Nursing*, 20, no. 1: 105–115.

Zabelina, D. L., Erickson, A. L., Kolotkin, R. L., and Crosby, R. D. (2009). The effect of age on weight-related quality of life in overweight and obese individuals. *Epidemiology*, 17, no. 7: 1410–1413.

Zhai, F., Wang, H., Du, S., He, Y., Wang, Z., Ge, K., and Popkin, B. M. (2009). Prospective study on nutrition transition in China. *Nutrition Review*, 67, suppl. 1: 556–561.

Zhang, Q., and Wang, Y. (2004). Socioeconomic inequality of obesity in the United States: Do gender, age, and ethnicity matter? *Social Science and Medicine*, 58, no. 6: 1171–1180.

Zhu, X., and Lee, C. (2008). Walkability and safety around elementary schools: Economic and ethnic disparities. *American Journal of Preventive Medicine*, 34, no. 4: 282–290.

Index